HAVE MILK, WILL TRAVEL

Adventures in Breastfeeding

Published by:
Demeter Press
140 Holland Street West
P. O. Box 13022
Bradford, ON L3Z 2Y5
Tel: (905) 775-9089
Email: info@demeterpress.org
Website: www.demeterpress.org

Demeter Press logo based on the sculpture "Demeter"
by Maria-Luise Bodirsky <www.keramik-atelier.bodirsky.de>

Front cover artwork: Rachel Epp Buller, "Untitled (sharing)," linoleum block print. Private collection.

Printed and Bound in Canada

Library and Archives Canada Cataloguing in Publication

        Have milk, will travel: adventures in breastfeeding / edited by Rachel
Epp Buller

        ISBN 978-1-927335-21-5

Cataloguing data available from Library and Archives Canada.

HAVE MILK, WILL TRAVEL

Adventures in Breastfeeding

edited by

Rachel Epp Buller

DEMETER PRESS, BRADFORD, ONTARIO

CONTENTS

CONTENTS

PREFACE

RACHEL EPP BULLER

W HEN IT COMES TO FEEDING BABIES, conventional wisdom tells us that "breast is best." Completely lacking in the how-and-why-to-nurse manuals, however, is an embrace of the comedy that lies just below the surface. Simply put, breastfeeding makes for some good laughs, so this book has been in the back of my mind ever since I nursed my own three children—on demand, on the go, through misadventures, and in all kinds of compromising situations.

As the stories collected here make clear, though, the fact that breastfeeding is not always easy comes as a surprise to most new mothers. Too much milk, not enough milk, trying to pump, dealing with infections and poor latches—who knew that it would be so complicated? Breastfeeding rates are on the rise: the most recent statistics show that nearly 77 percent of American mothers initiate breastfeeding, but the fact that only 45 percent still nurse at all after six months suggests that many moms lack support. And we don't make it easy on each other: we might be bad mothers if we *don't* nurse, for whatever reason, or if we nurse for *too long*, and yet breastfeeding in public often results in social discomfort and negative reactions.

Blame and guilt help nothing. Our bodies do not always work as we expect them to, and breastfeeding does not always go as planned. What will help, I hope, is the support of mother-writers who have been there and survived, who now know that mothering and nursing come in all shapes and sizes, in all kinds of experiences and outcomes.

I give thanks for everyone who submitted stories for consideration. I am awed by the honesty with which writers shared their experiences, whether joyous, painful, or just painfully embarrassing. Special thanks go to Sarah Pinneo, who read early drafts of the book proposal and gave such thoughtful feedback; to Andrea O'Reilly, who believed in the book; to Cheryl Petran, whose enthusiasm made possible a collaboration with The Pump Station & Nurtury; to Tim, who supported breastfeeding even when it cut him out of the picture; and to my children, who first taught me about life as the one-stop milk shop.

FOREWORDS:
A TALE OF TWO LACTATION CONSULTANTS

CORKY HARVEY AND WENDY HALDEMAN

*S*O *YOU THINK YOU WANT TO BREASTFEED? An honest mother might tell you: it was the best of times, it was the worst of times. Corky Harvey and Wendy Haldeman have seen it all. Having worked as nurses in maternal and newborn health, as Lamaze teachers, and as lactation consultants, Wendy and Corky founded The Pump Station & Nurtury in California over 25 years ago in order to provide a much-needed baby boot camp in breastfeeding and new parent resources. What began as a home office has expanded to a thriving business with multiple locations and thousands of clients.*

Corky Harvey:
   Early in my career, a pediatrician who I worked for always introduced me as a "lactating" consultant—even when I had long since weaned my last child. I never got tired of the joke because, honestly, when you work in the world of breastfeeding, you are already in the center of a "funny" occupation.
   Don't get me wrong: I couldn't be any more passionate about my dedication to helping women successfully nurse their babies and to changing the norm in our culture from formula feeding to breastfeeding. But there is something inherently humorous in any job that gets this kind of response, over and over again:
   "So, what do you do for a living?"
   "I'm a lactation consultant."
   "Uhm—a what?"
   "I help women with breastfeeding."

1

"You're kidding right? Women actually need help with that?" Another common response—always from men: "Hey, I'm looking for extra work. Need an assistant? (Nudge, nudge, wink, wink)."

I've had chances to give back the same kind of remarks: at a recent high school reunion, after describing my occupation to an audience of almost a hundred of my classmates, I looked right in the face of one of my favorite guy friends and said, "Hey Mike, just like you, breasts are my life." It was a hilarious moment.

You can't work in a job like this, meeting so many mothers and hearing about their experiences, without getting a Thousand and One Nights' worth of great stories about funny, often embarrassing moments. The accidental "flashing" tales can be the funniest and most memorable. My niece had her two-week old baby in her arms when she answered the door to receive a package from the UPS man. She didn't realize until the door was closed again that one bra "flap" was completely down.

A surgeon that I worked with a few years ago once flew to San Francisco to speak at a conference, leaving her young, nursing baby at home. She had notified the conference organizers that she would need to pump before her lecture, but when she arrived at the airport, time was short. The organizers had sent two young men to the airport to pick her up. One opened the door and offered her a seat in the back. She refused, and slid instead into the front passenger seat. She whipped out her breast pump, plugged it into the lighter outlet, and pumped all the way to the venue. I can only imagine the conversation that ensued between those two after she left the vehicle—and probably over beers at the local bar for many weeks after that.

My husband gave me a wonderful, surprise fortieth birthday party at an up-scale Chinese restaurant. The cake was a huge masterpiece: two gorgeous breasts complete with areola and nipples. While keeping their professional demeanor, the poor waiters' faces were a treat to watch as they searched for the perfect places to "stick" the candles. The cheers of the crowd were rich.

We have good friends that I helped with breastfeeding years ago. Every time I see them, the father's greeting to me is the same—a salute, with his right hand over his left breast, and a wink.

Sometimes humor is a defense, since some people still don't understand the importance of breastfeeding for an infant's health and the bond it creates between mother and baby. Things have improved since the day my first child was breastfeeding, but women still often feel judged and criticized—even by close family members. When my first baby was six weeks old, people would sometimes look at me and say, in a condescending tone, "How long are you gonna breastfeed that baby?" I already had my snappy answer ready: "Oh, I'll wean him before he goes to college." And I did.

My three children have never known life without breastfeeding; it has always seemed completely normal to them. Hearing me on the phone dealing with breastfeeding issues gave them the ability to answer questions about sore nipples and engorgement from an early age. I was in a grocery store with my two oldest kids, ages four and six months, when a baby further up the aisle started wailing loudly. The mother was trying her best to console her child as we passed. My matter-of-fact little boy looked straight up at her and said, "Lady, why don't you breastfeed your baby?" He already knew one solution for calming an infant. At age three, my youngest son was producing a puppet show from behind the living room couch where I stored large rental breast pumps. He and his friend were a bit too short and needed a boost. I heard my little guy say to his friend, "Here Danny, just stand up on this breast pump." It sure made me smile.

My daughter is an über-nurser and now a lactation professional, too. She and her still-nursing toddler flew to her brother's graduation in Atlanta. As the family walked around the campus or toured the town, her son would decide it was time for a snack and would look around for a place for his mom to sit down. When he found just the right spot, he'd point toward it with one hand while making the sign for milk with his other. It made us laugh until we cried.

Breastfeeding is not necessarily easy and requires strong resolve and much support. My favorite part of the job is facilitating the Breastfeeding Support Groups at The Pump Station & Nurtury. Here, moms come together with their young babies to ask questions and "hang out" with others who are in the same place in life. It is today's *kaffeklatsch* and it's wonderful. There are always tears from the exhausted and overwhelmed, encouragement from everyone, and lots and lots of laughter. The tough, embarrassing, and funny situations these new mothers share help everyone leave feeling renewed and ready to carry on for another week. Plans are made to meet for the mommy movies, lunch, or walks in the park. Friendships are formed for life. Babies are so adorable and amazing—but mothering and breastfeeding can be difficult, lonely, and even boring at times. Keeping it enjoyable and lighthearted helps to make it a richer experience and keep it doable. In the scheme of things, breastfeeding our little ones is such a brief span in our lives and it should be experienced to the fullest. I love what I do and I love all the crazy, fun experiences that I get to hear every day of my life from all the wonderful moms that I'm blessed to meet. Laughter truly remains the best medicine.

Wendy Haldeman:

It is not necessary to possess a sense of humor to succeed at breastfeeding. But having been a mother, grandmother and lactation consultant for twenty-six years, I would suggest that humor definitely helps to get a harried breastfeeding mom over a rough patch. Motherhood is challenging, to say the least. The responsibilities can be overwhelming. Laughter can be invaluable when trying to surmount all the challenges that parenting and breastfeeding can present. Experienced mothers have much to share with new women just beginning to take on this role, and amusing stories are a wonderful way to endear us to one another.

As one of the founding members of The Pump Station & Nurtury, I have plenty of pumping and nursing adventures to share. Many years ago, I worked with a new mom, Jennifer, who was going to be her sister's matron of honor. The wedding was scheduled six weeks after Jennifer delivered her first baby. Many hours of preparation went into designing a plan of action so that Jennifer would be able to perform her wedding duties as well as care for her new baby. She had scheduled her pumping session to occur just before she had to enter the church. Everything was going perfectly until she stood up and promptly dumped the entire bottle of expressed milk down her dress. Nothing to do but pick up her bouquet and proceed down the aisle.

Working outside the home and continuing to maintain a milk supply presents many challenges. My sister loves to tell the story of how she had returned to work after her second baby. She is a C.E.O. for a corporation and was scheduled to make a major presentation to her board of directors her first day back at work. Stressed and harried, she left home without any breast pads. Five minutes prior to the beginning of her presentation, she began to leak copious amounts of milk onto her silk blouse. She grabbed her suit jacket to cover the wet spots and marched into the conference room, only to discover that the air conditioning was broken. So, for the next two hours she proceeded to leak and sweat profusely.

My daughters have been subjected to many of my adventures over the years. They remember vividly when one day we were approached by one of my clients. She was overjoyed to have run into me as she related that she was worried about one of her nipples. She pulled up her shirt and pulled down her bra and asked me what I thought. I responded that I thought we should find a more appropriate location to talk about her nipple that was not the parking lot of Toys "R" Us!

Nursing toddlers can often create memorable situations. I have a friend and colleague who many years ago liked to frequent a topless beach with her family. She, her husband, and two-and-a-half-year-old son had made their way down to this beach on a gloriously warm summer day. After setting up the chairs, towels, and umbrella, the toddler was ensconced with his sand toys. A young woman, perhaps around eighteen years of age, also made her way to said beach. She placed her towel onto the sand, removed her top, stretched out on her towel on her back and fell asleep. The toddler watched this young woman for a few minutes and then left his sand castle, walked over and promptly latched onto her breast. I guess he was looking for a little variety. The young woman was truly shocked—she leapt up, grabbed her belongings, and was never seen again.

I have facilitated numerous breastfeeding support groups over the past twenty years and have laughed and cried at so many wonderful and touching stories that mothers have shared with one another. The neophyte struggling with her new role as mother can find tremendous comfort in learning about the trials other women have dealt with and won. Laughter is uplifting and healing. We can all benefit from sharing stories and anecdotes. This book is full of memorable tales of the breastfeeding mother. Grab a comfortable chair, put your feet up, and prepare to enjoy yourself.

BOOBY TRAPPED

JENNA McCARTHY

WHEN YOU'RE AN ON-AIR RADIO PERSONALITY—and your co-host is a guy—you live by a simple motto: Everything's a bit. (And a "bit" is anything that makes for amusing radio banter.) Like the time I drove away from a gas pump with the nozzle still nestled in my car's tank? That became the ever-popular "Dumber than Jenna" game—where callers who confessed to any move more idiotic than mine were rewarded with concert tickets or a station t-shirt. *Everything's a bit.*

Despite the fact that he'd be running the show solo during my upcoming maternity leave, my co-host was oddly delighted when I told him I was expecting my first child. And not because we'd been friends for years or even because of that whole "miracle of life" business. To hell with all of that! His interest in my condition was limited to how best to exploit the crazy cravings, blossoming belly and porn-star boobs that would soon fill our studio. My bump was the Ultimate Bit. He began taking copious notes involving potty pools (How Many Times an Hour Will Jenna Have to Pee?), guess-the-week's-weight-gain games, and Make Me Gag competitions. The potential bits were countless.

I trundled through the months and actually enjoyed sharing my daily discomforts with thousands of faceless listeners. An offhand remark about heartburn, nausea, or spontaneously bleeding gums would spawn dozens of sympathetic calls. When my due date came and went, I was admitted to the hospital for an induction. (Apparently the baby in my stomach was growing to the size of a nice Thanksgiving turkey, and the wary doctors wanted her out before the Jaws of Life became necessary; believe me when I tell you I did not put up a fight.) At one point in the delivery room, between raging contractions, my cell phone rang.

"Hello?" I growled into it, heee-heee-hooo-hoooing through gritted teeth. I couldn't have told you if it was midnight on a Monday or high noon on Halloween, much less why I thought it necessary to answer my damned phone. I blame the drugs.

"Hey Jenna, you're on the air!" my co-host chuckled in his velvety Moviefone voice.

I can't recall exactly what I said in reply, but I'd bet good money it wasn't something you'd want to repeat to your sweet old grandmother.

Within days I had my shiny new baby at home with me, where I spent long hours staring at her angelic face and marveling at the fact that I'd built an entire person inside of my very own body. Also I made milk. Gallons of it. At first I dispensed all of it directly into my daughter's hungry mouth, but soon I realized that I had better start stockpiling the "liquid gold"—as we called it—for when I went back to work.

To say that I wasn't a fan of pumping breast milk is like saying syrup-dipped marshmallows are a little on the sweet side. When childless friends would ask what it was like, the same words always leapt to mind: Unnatural. Uncomfortable. Awkward. Endless. But breast is best, and nobody was going to accuse *me* of giving my kid sloppy, synthetic seconds if I could help it.

So I'd sit and be milked by a machine for several collective hours a day. It took my pump a good fifteen to twenty minutes to drain each teat—*each time*—and I found it not a little disconcerting that I would consistently get three times more milk from the same overachieving side. My freezer began to look like a warped Warhol tribute to motherhood.

Although I was back at work—in body at least—I also was suffering from the sort of Mommy Brain Syndrome that led me to do things like leave my car keys in my underwear drawer and drive away with the house phone stashed neatly in my purse. Which is the only way I can explain how I didn't see this next bit (pun very much intended) coming.

"I need to go pump," I announced to my co-host, taking off my headphones. I had been watching the schedule for a break in the on-air action, and we were looking at a fifteen minute stretch of commercials. It wasn't ideal, but it was enough time to at least take the edge off.

"Take your cell phone," he replied.

"Why would I need..." I began, and then I stopped. *He wanted me to do this—whip out my naked boobs and have them be suckled by an appliance—on the air.*

"Come on, Jenna," he pleaded. "Everything's a bit, remember?"

I shuffled to the ladies room, clutching my unwieldy pump bag protectively to my massive cleavage. Just as I had hooked myself up, my cell phone rang. The pump wheezed and pulled, moaned and sucked.

"Hello?" I said with the casual, breezy air of a woman who *wasn't sitting cupping her topless breasts while thousands of strangers were picturing her doing exactly that.*

"What's going on?" announcer-guy asked with annoying nonchalance.

Wheeze, pull, moan, suck.

"Oh, you know," I bellowed over the echoing machine. "Just whipping up a little dinner in here."

I listened to the taped show later, and it was actually pretty funny. And I consoled myself with the reminder that at least I worked in radio—and not TV. My favorite email of the day read simply this: "Thanks for the mammaries."

UNDIGNIFIED POSITIONS

BETH WINEGARNER

IT'S FOUR O'CLOCK IN THE MORNING, and I'm leaning over the kitchen table, topless, with my breasts soaking in mismatched mixing bowls filled with salty hot water. I'm reading a glossy fashion magazine while I soak, as though I were relaxing in a spa somewhere, waiting for a massage or a pedicure. In reality, though, I'm watching the clock, because after I've soaked for 15 minutes I will cozy up with the breast pump—the one whose rhythmic wheeze, I swear, has started whispering to me in the middle of nights like these.

Let me back up: My daughter was born in March of 2009, and within the first eight weeks of her life, I fought mastitis three times. Each time the treatment was the same: moist heat every two hours, followed by nursing or the pump, not to mention up to two weeks of antibiotics (plus probiotics, to keep my nether regions from turning into a yeast factory). It was as though the Universe said, "You know, mothering a newborn just isn't challenging enough for you. I know breast-feeding is like learning a foreign language overnight, and the sleep deprivation is worse than a bad acid trip, but let's see how you handle *this*."

Before my daughter was born, I learned plenty about breastfeeding. But nobody told me about mastitis, the breast infection that indicates that breastfeeding has gone somehow awry. They didn't mention how it makes you feel like your breasts are lit matches, your body's been tumble-dried, and your mind is melting.

I'm not entirely sure what's happening that first time, when I wake up with two hot, swollen, red-streaked breasts and a fever like I imagine comes with some exotic jungle disease. But exotic jungle diseases come with exotic jungle vacations, right? And hospital beds with soft, cool sheets, and nurses sponging you down with cold water while murmuring soothing phrases to you in their native language as you drift in and out of consciousness. This fever—with a hungry, crying three-week-old baby rooting at my incandescent boobs—isn't like that at all.

So we—my partner, daughter and I—schlep to UC San Francisco Medical Center's Labor & Delivery unit. A stern New Yorker midwife enters the curtain surrounding my bed, opens my gown, and places her cool hands on my breasts. "Oh, my," she says, reacting to my unlucky bosom. "How old is your baby?"

"Three weeks," I say.

"Yep, right on schedule," she says. "Most moms who develop mastitis do it right around the three-week mark."

She runs hot water over a pair of hospital towels and presses them to my chest, but they cool quickly, dribbling cold water into my lap. I'm going to look like I've peed myself, but a number of nurses have come and gone from my room, so the idea of dignity seems very remote just now. Meanwhile, the midwife disappears and returns with a long tube capped with a cotton swab. "I'm so sorry," she says.

"Sorry for—Ow!"

Before I can ask why she's apologizing, she wraps her fingers around my blazing areola and squeezes, coaxing milk out of the nipple. She swabs the milk into the tube, hoping that if they test it, they can identify which bacteria, precisely, has come to visit.

The midwife and nurses disappear for a while. I have been given freshly wetted towels with which to soothe my aching tits. Meanwhile, my partner is giving our daughter a tour of the cramped hospital room. Since she was born at home, it's her first time in one, and he's showing her how the beds go up and down, pointing out the blood-pressure gear, the sink, the IV poles. Being just three weeks old, she's a bit wide-eyed, both oblivious and agreeable to her circumstances. He photographs her next to a ziplock bag with a biohazard logo printed on it—and then changes her diaper, depositing the soiled nappy in the bag. After that, we breastfeed awkwardly on the narrow hospital bed.

From there, we go to Walgreens to fill my antibiotics prescription. By the time we leave the hospital it's quite late, and one of the only 24-hour Walgreens in San Francisco is in the heart of the Castro, the city's gay mecca. This is my favorite drugstore in the whole city. Walgreens always tailors its window displays to its clientele, and this one includes leopard-print pajamas, satin slippers, yoga mats, and sweaters for tiny dogs. As I sit and wait for my medicine, my partner carries our daughter up and down the aisles, dazzling her with endless varieties of medicine, kitchen utensils, and questionable snack foods. Next to me, gay couples clutch each other's hands and pore over the impressively large array of lube and condoms.

Back at home, I realize I need to come up with an alternative to the hot-towel thing. Not only do they cool off quickly, but they're messy. That's how I come up with the idea of soaking in mixing-bowls. I'm not crazy about being in this undignified position for ten to fifteen minutes, every two hours. My partner, on the other hand, loves it: it gives him the opportunity to goose me every time he walks by.

Mastitis has encroached on our lives at a time when we are planning to attend a panel discussion on the topic of infant vaccinations. Due to the outcry over supposed links between autism and vaccines, the topic of inoculation is a touchy one in our liberal city. We want to make an informed choice. Somehow, attending a panel featuring a couple of health-care workers, a homeopath, and a mom who didn't vaccinate her kids, seems like the best way to go about doing this.

But I'm way, way too sick to go. My partner suggests going on his own, leaving me alone with the baby for the first time while he treks across town. I should be thanking him for gathering information that will help us make the first of many difficult decisions about our daughter's health. Instead, I burst into tears.

"What if my fever gets worse?" I ask him. "What if the baby does something unexpected, like poops her diaper or cries? What if burglars break into the house, gather up our valuables, and then point and laugh at my feeble attempt to mother a newborn while fevered out of my gourd?"

Okay, none of that actually came out of my mouth. But it did cross my mind.

Instead, I say, "Please don't go. Please, please, please. I can't do this."

"You'll be fine," he says. "It's only for a few hours."

He stocks the bedroom with thermoses of cold water to drink, trail mix, and other snacks. He sets me up with the baby in my nursing chair, next to the breast pump and heating pad. He kisses me on the head and wishes me luck.

Soon after he leaves, the baby wakes. She begins rooting, looking for a spot of milk. I latch her on. She nurses contentedly for a few minutes, and then begins to doze again. I take a sip of cold water and nibble on a little trail mix. *This isn't so bad*, I think. *She can just sleep, and he'll only be gone a couple of hours. I can do this.*

That's when I hear a weird noise in the hall, just outside the bedroom door. I snap my head in the direction of the sound—a kind of scrubbing shuffle. Through the doorway I watch as our cat drags her ass down the hall, crazed look in her eyes, paws scrabbling frantically. It's as though she's trying to escape some fiery hellhound, except her hindquarters are velcroed to the floor. That's when I notice the lengthening brown trail on the carpet behind her. It's no hellhound, but a piece of poop that has stuck to her butt after a visit to the litter box. Now it's streaked down the hallway, and here I am, alone with a sleeping newborn and a raging breast infection.

I start to cry. And laugh.

It wakes the baby.

LIQUID GOLD

SARAH PINNEO

B Y THE TIME I READ THE PAMPHLET, I was already sold
on the idea of breastfeeding.

As I trundled towards my ninth pregnant month, the
chorus of boob propaganda seemed to rise to a fevered pitch. It
came from all sides—from well-meaning friends, from scientific
studies, and finally from a pamphlet in the obstetrician's office.
But of course I would give breastfeeding a try—to stimulate my
baby's immune system, to burn off pregnancy fat, to decrease
the chances of my baby ever facing allergies, diabetes, obesity,
lower I.Q. Apparently there was nothing that breastfeeding
couldn't cure.

Still, as I scanned this list of tantalizing benefits, the last
exuberant bullet point caught my eye.

"And last but not least, breastfeeding is free!"

The fact that the "equipment" was bought and paid for
was indeed a perk. My inner cheapskate couldn't help but be
excited by the savings. After all, our apartment was rapidly
filling with expensive baby accoutrements. There were ergo-
nomically correct bouncy seats, organic cotton onesies and an
intimidating stroller. Saving money became more attractive by
the minute. And baby formula is surprisingly expensive—about
$0.22 per ounce in liquid form.

I've drunk wines cheaper than that. Many times.

So in the happy fog of my first hours of motherhood, and
with the help of a nurse, I did precisely what was expected of
me. Eight-pound, round-cheeked Jack was popped onto my

left nipple, which he took without hesitation.

"Congratulations!" the nurse gushed. "He has a terrific latch."

The euphoria lasted only a few seconds, because that's when the pain set in. Jack did indeed have a terrific latch. Terrific for *him*. For me, it felt as though I'd been munched by a barracuda. The pain and bleeding began immediately, and did not relent. By the time he was a week old, every feeding brought me to tears. But I was resolute. So the tiny tube of lanolin ointment that the hospital had sent home with me was used up, and my husband ran to the drug store for a new one. At $10, it was a bargain.

For support, I called upon my wonderful friend Barbara, who had once let slip that she'd had a lot of trouble at first with nursing. I described to her all of my various miseries. "There's the bleeding, of course," I told her. "And I'm so tense that I've hunched my back too. I just can't get comfortable."

"Oh! You need My Brest Friend," she said.

"Who?"

"It's a nursing pillow with back support. It saved my life. You could also try nipple shields—soft plastic cups which stand between your nipple and the baby's mouth."

I thanked her tearfully, and once again my husband was dispatched into the great big world, this time in search of an embarrassingly named cushion, at $40, and nipple shields for $7.99.

As I awaited his return, it occurred to me that breastfeeding was no longer free. Were I a fly upon the wall at the very aptly named *Buy Buy Baby* store, I could have at least heard the poor man clear his throat and ask the salesperson for nipple shields. I could have recouped something of my money at least in entertainment value.

As it happened, little Jack wasn't wild about the nipple shields. I threw them away after just a few tries.

Yet I soldiered on. Things improved, if only slightly. I ordered two nursing bras ($60), and a nursing top ($39 plus shipping).

I wanted to become one of those mothers who could plop right down on the park bench and nurse anywhere. But my troubles persisted. As we rolled toward the end of week two, I finally did the smart thing. I called a lactation consultant.

I had never *met* one before—or even heard of lactation consultants. And Ilana did not disappoint. She wore flowing skirts, a romantic hat, and a calm demeanor. My husband still refers to her as Ilana the Good Witch. Whether or not all lactation consultants resemble earthy fairy godmothers, I cannot say. But boy, was she helpful.

"May I touch your breast?" she asked quietly.

"Go for it." When your nipples resemble weeping sores, modesty actually hurts more than nudity before strangers.

"Ouch, yes," she said gently. "We will have to improve your swing."

"Pardon?"

But I hadn't misheard her. The lesson that followed—careful instructions on how to latch the baby's mouth so far onto the breast that my nipple was closer to his epiglottis than his Fangs of Doom—was rather like a golf lesson that I'd once been forced to take for a corporate outing.

"A proper latch," Ilana the Good Witch explained, "is all in the wrist."

"Oh!" I felt the difference immediately. "You've really jammed him on there."

In her characteristic hush she delivered a line of wisdom that my husband and I would quote for weeks afterward. "No one has ever been killed by a breast."

So successful was Ilana at reducing my pain, I didn't even begrudge her the $175 fee. And likewise, the hospital quality breast pump she recommended, at $150 to *rent*, was a life saver too. But then there were the bottles—the very ones I'd expected to avoid buying in the first place—at $26 for a "starter set."

"Free" breastfeeding had by then cost me over $500, though I won't bother to add the cost of the cabbage leaves that Ilana the Good Witch recommended wearing in my bra for just one day, as a natural pain reliever. Their cost was small. Especially since my husband made a lovely coleslaw from the leftovers.

Breastfeeding, I'm told, sets up the baby and mother for life with a host of benefits—medical, nutritional and psychological. Now that my son is older I'm sure our healthy start together will pay dividends for years to come.

But like any good investment, just be prepared to find that there are a few unadvertised fees along the way.

MILK WITH A MAYAN KING

ALERIA JENSEN

It was supposed to be your pilgrimage, after all.
For so long the dream of that jungle,
ruins rising through vines, stonework, tombs,
name a mystery on the tongue—*Palenque*.
And now the time to meet it, its own mystery—
maternity leave.

The first night—a fan that barely turned,
side-nursing on a single sagging bed.
Body sticking to baby in wet heat and tears.
Why did you bring an infant,
what were you thinking?
Dad sleeping soundly in his own bed.

Next day there are bugs, temperatures
near one hundred, and a small creature
who only wants to nurse. Nevertheless,
you wait in the dust for the bus, baby in Bjorn,
morning buzzing with green light and fire.

Finally, you step into the clearing—ancient
courtyard where limestone soars into a blue
universe, where the Tomb of the Red Queen lies
buried in jade and obsidian, sprinkled with cinnabar,
her body beneath an eight ton sarcophagus within
a temple of painstaking proportions.

Here, your life stills...

...for a microsecond, because your son
is wailing. You nurse under a *ceiba* tree
while local guides stop to tell tourists
how its trunk gives life, its roots speak
to the dead, its spines pierce Mayan fingers,
fertilizing the earth with blood.

You never imagined this heat, nor that
you wouldn't explore every pyramid.
You nurse, pace, sing lullabies—he bawls.
Finally, there's nothing to do but seek
darkness—duck into opening, into
passageway, into chamber while sweat
greases your arms and simmers
between your breasts.

You collapse on stone rectangle
in the dim hallway where again you offer
milk as tourists file by, where again
you are the spectacle. Spit-up sours
thick air, but you breathe it, surrendering,
as you must, to the improbable present.

Eavesdropping, you learn that
you are nursing on the bed of Lord
Pakal, ruler of Palenque, King.
That his bed was layered with the pelts
of jaguars, softened by feather pillows,
that he lay cooled by palm fronds,
fanned by the hands of slaves.

What would he think, the King? Is it profane
to nurse on a sacred bed, or, is it, in fact,

absolutely perfect? You have to laugh
for the wildness of it all—his home, your dream,
his leisure, your pain, his kingdom, your milk,
the silken strand stitching it whole,
the invisible thread of spirit through stone.

So this is how the pilgrimage ends:
clutching the one who requires so much of you,
deep inside the palace,
deep inside the blaze of motherhood,
just where you were meant to be,
in the heart of it all, sunk
to your knees
in love.

MY BROKEN BOOBS

JILL NEUMANN

WHEN IT COMES TO BABIES, there are just *so* many choices. Co-sleeping or crib? Disposables or cloth? Breastmilk or formula? Before I had a child, I always thought that I would breastfeed. All the research said it was best, provided a special bonding time unique to only you *and* it was free. I especially liked the free part. Nursing, I decided, was the best choice for me.

I also wrongly assumed that it *was* a choice.

So when I welcomed a daughter in June of 2011, I was mentally ready to go. I had read the articles, talked to friends and bought the pump. When my hopes for an all-natural, drug-free birth (HA HA HA HA!) went down the drain after too many hours in labor with not enough results, my kiddo was born by c-section, face-up and blue.

She was whisked away to the NICU where she spent five days working out a few issues. In the meantime, I recovered from a hellish labor and surgery in my hospital room three floors above her. Definitely not the birth story I had imagined. I was wheeled down to visit her every three hours for feedings. It was there in the NICU that I nursed my daughter for the very first time. She latched on fabulously. No problems there! The problem was, she was getting very little milk.

The nurses told me this was normal and that my milk should be coming in any day now. They advised me to pump to help things along. So I pumped. And pumped. And pumped some more. Each time, the small cylindrical bottles remained nearly empty. Again they told me this was normal and that it takes some women a little longer for their milk to fully come in.

So I kept pumping and was able to eke out about an ounce from each breast. And every three hours, I carried my measly ounces of breast milk down to the NICU and carefully attached the nipple, as if it were a magical, rare serum. Priceless. Unicorn tears. I gave her the tiny bottle, imagining that these few drops for which I had pumped for *so* long would hit her tongue, roll down her throat and suddenly, beams of light would shoot out her ten tiny fingers and ten tiny toes. Just like all the books said, breast milk *was* amazing! I could hear her brain cells multiplying, especially the math ones. She opened her blue eyes and had x-ray vision. Looking down at my angel, I wondered how I would teach her to control her super powers as a young child. Punching through her kindergarten walls. Would the other children ostracize her because she was so much faster and smarter than they? These were things we'd just have to deal with when the time came, I thought, smiling down at her.

And then the nurse handed me the second tiny bottle. Until my milk came in, I had to supplement her feedings with— GASP!—formula. The F-word. She took the bottle with equal vigor as the breast milk and then came back for seconds. Oh no, I thought. What if she gets used to the formula before my own milk comes in? I could hear her brain cells shrinking and deforming. Her eyes glazed over and she stared off at nothing in particular. Would she be the kid in class who always stuck things in her nose? *That* kid? I could hear her now, coming home from school saying, "Mommy, I want to be a reality TV star."

Damn you, formula! Come on, boobs! Work!

I pumped harder. More frequently. I talked to the lactation specialists. I started taking Fenugreek and Blessed Thistle herbal supplements. Drinking special herbal teas. I nursed. I pumped. Friends offered advice, ranging from yoga positions to skin-to-skin contact to "just relax." Still, only a few drops were left at the bottom of the bottle after all of our collective efforts.

After five days in the NICU, I could finally bring my new baby home. She was healthy and beautiful and perfect. My boobs, however, were still big, lousy disappointments.

I was a big, lousy disappointment.

One bizarre thought kept passing through my brain. I couldn't help but imagine that it was 10,000 B.C. and here I was, in my cave. The baby's corner had been all decked out in the softest regional animal pelts and the surrounded walls had all been painted with the most colorful dancing bison and spear-wielding figures. My pet dinosaur had been sleeping with the baby's loincloth for a week now to get him used to her smells. (I know that's not historically accurate, but it's my fantasy and I can have a pet dinosaur if I want.) Everything was perfect! Yet all this meant nothing if I could not do the one thing that she needed most. I couldn't feed her! Without my milk, she simply wouldn't survive long enough to enjoy her mobile of dried flowers hung from the stalactites above. She would never gather her first berry nor make her first fire. I realized that it wasn't, in fact, 10,000 B.C. We had modern medicine and formula and ways to foil stupid, uncooperating nature. But that wasn't the point.

The point was that I was a failure at the single thing that was most important to me. I was a failure as a mother.

Maybe it was the hormones or the sleep-deprivation, or perhaps simply my stubbornness, but I wouldn't give up. I couldn't accept that my body was just not going to produce milk. I kept trying. Kiddo was a champ at latching and sucked unbelievably hard. Maybe she was getting more milk than I thought she was? How could one really tell, anyway? My god, does she suck hard! My nipples hurt, but that was normal, right? I kept at it.

On the fourth day home from the hospital, I was nursing Kiddo in bed. She had sucked for a long time before I balanced her on my lap with one hand and burped her with the other. One good burp. And then it happened. My tiny baby projectile-vomited all over me, all over herself, all over the bed. A massive amount. My brain processed this quickly and realized that this was not your normal post-feeding spit-up. It was red. Blood red.

Something was very wrong.

In the car speeding to the hospital, I tried to focus. She's going to be okay, I thought. She's going to be fine. But the terror was beyond anything I had experienced. Were these the quiet moments before the storm? Before one's world is turned upside down with a horrible, life-altering diagnosis? Would there be hospital stays? Procedures? Grim diagnoses? Would people say, "Did you hear about Jill's baby? It's so sad." Was this the moment that everything changes?

Oh please let her be okay. Please. I'll do anything. Please just let her be okay. None of it matters anymore, not the formula, not the soft animal pelts, not the future love of reality TV shows. Even if she sticks things in her nose as a child, *especially* if she sticks things in her nose as a child. Just please be okay. Please oh please, oh please *let my baby be okay.*

At the hospital they ran some tests. The doctor finally came in the room with the results.

"She's going to be okay," he said. "It's not her blood. It's *your* blood. STOP BREASTFEEDING."

I sat there stunned. As it turned out, Kiddo had a damn good latch after all. Though I had no evidence of cracks or bleeding, she had been sucking so hard that she was sucking my own blood. My baby was a vampire.

We went home. I zipped up my expensive breast pump and put it in the garage. I threw out the Fenugreek and the breast milk storage freezer bags and the nursing bras and the nipple cream (okay, I kept the nipple cream). I microwaved Kiddo a bottle of formula. She happily gobbled it up.

My boobs eventually completely dried up and deflated. I had lost the breastfeeding battle. Turns out, it wasn't a choice after all.

And, if I were to be completely honest, there was a tiny part of me that was relieved. Breastfeeding is *hard*. Though I was ready for the commitment that it took, part of me was glad that I had a reason that would be seen as valid by most all mothers why I formula-fed. "Well, at least you *tried*," the hardcore Earth Mothers would say. "Meh, you're better off," the Team Formula moms would advise.

As for me? I think about how I was given formula as a baby, as were many children of the '70s and '80s. And I turned out pretty okay, right? *Right?* As I watch my now-toddler name all of the colors of the rainbow and then try to jam the entire remote control into her mouth, I realize she's going to be just fine. Because in the end, it really doesn't matter what you choose, or even if it *was* a choice or not. We put far too much pressure on ourselves to do what's Right, even when there is no such thing as Right to begin with. What matters is not your best laid plans. Not your stupid, broken boobs. What matters is that smile. That laugh. That she's happy and healthy and on her way to sticking things up her nose and living to tell about it.

BREAST IS BEST

MOSA MAXWELL-SMITH

IN THE NINTH GRADE, Brian Cabrillo and I went to the beach at night and got to second base. He asked to have my black mesh bra with the satin trim as a souvenir. Despite his impassioned pleas, I declined. My rationale was that if I gave him my bra, he would see the tag, which said not only, "Victoria's Secret," but "34A." As if somehow his fast, needy hands had not felt my Size A in the flesh, I knew the tag would be the thing to announce my shamefully small cup size. Later, as I draped the loosely fitting mesh across my chest and fastened it on the tightest setting, I praised myself for narrowly escaping revealing the truth about my breasts, or lack thereof.

Years after Brian and I broke up, after suffering the torture of my mom altering my bikini top in high school to make it smaller, and watching various hip, vintage dresses sag and droop across my chest, I still hadn't come to terms with my less than ample bosom. I held out hope throughout my teenage years: maybe I was just a late bloomer; maybe, despite the fact that I had started my period at age twelve, my boobs were just taking their time.

By my twenty-first birthday, I had convinced myself that waiting any longer would be bordering on insanity—it was time to take action. I invested in padded bras and some foul-smelling cream and supplements from the new-fangled Internet. Together, the bras and the cream worked to make me smell like the rancid rejects from a vitamin store; the cream smelled on its own, but the padding made me sweat more and amplified the already pungent odor. Needless to say, the only thing that increased in size was my shame about my just-as-small-but-now-super-stinky breasts.

After spending the better part of my twenties with my breasts encased in enough water and foam and "miracle gel" to protect them from a nuclear holocaust, I pulled out the big guns, so to speak. Afraid of surgery, I opted instead to spend thousands of dollars on giant plastic domes that fit over my breasts and attached to a special vacuum that was to pull, pull, pull my breasts to their new larger cup size. Yes, I bought that. During the three-month process, I woke everyday with sweaty plastic domes and swollen breasts. I delighted in my buxomness each morning, but by nightfall, like balloons at the end of a county fair, my bosoms were a droopy, depressing reminder of the buoyant joy that had once been. The effects were not lasting.

Just shy of my thirty-second birthday, I made the ultimate commitment to natural breast enhancement. Research told me that only one small injection would increase my breast size significantly and have lasting results that I could prolong with proper maintenance. How could I go wrong? I got pregnant.

Almost instantly, I felt my chest swell. Perhaps it was the increased intake of ice cream that commenced upon conception or the pride at becoming a new mama—maybe there was a hormone or two. The precise reason mattered not; my method was working. Finally! A natural breast enhancement system with proven results. Take that, cosmetic surgeons!

There's a picture of me on the New Year's Eve when I was five months pregnant. I am wearing a fantastically low-cut dress, bosoms pouring out the top, threatening to expose themselves fully to the other guests in attendance. Among its other merits, the dress did an excellent job of camouflaging my also expanding belly and hips—a small (err, not so small) price to pay for boobs, I say!

As my body continued to expand throughout pregnancy, I focused on the boob part—the weight of my breasts against my ribs, my t-shirts stretched taut against my chest, the shallow pool of cleavage where perspiration and sandwich crumbs could collect. Late in my pregnancy, I remember bragging unabashedly about the fact that a large piece of popcorn had fallen into my bra and gotten lost there for several hours. I didn't even notice it because my breasts were like a large mountain range. How could I be expected to keep track of a piddle-y piece of popcorn without GPS, or, at the very least, a meager map?

Nearly at term, fantasizing wildly about how my already gargantuan breasts might further develop with the help of a suckling infant, I got a bit of a reality check. Standing in a large group of other pregnant women and some new moms, one of my friends, looking directly at my Dolly Parton-esque rack said, "Wow, your boobs are really ... (giant? nicely-shaped? voluptuous? I thought) ... small for someone who is as pregnant as you are." I suppose size is relative; in their new "huge" state, my boobs were barely pushing the limits of a B cup. Well, in my world, "B" stands for Beautiful, Bountiful, Big Breasts! I was proud of my chest for the first time in my life, regardless of what others thought of it.

All through my adolescence, I had tried to hide my breasts from clumsy fondlers—lovers is too strong a word, methinks. I guided hands away from my small breasts hovering in their padded caves. Now, with a lovely fifteen month-old daughter suckling daily, I am still relishing my huge-to-me boobs. Realizing their ephemeral nature, I am embracing every moment of my large-breastedness. I nurse in public, thinking nothing of whipping out a breast at a restaurant or a public park. I wear push-up bras with low cut tops. I delight in photographs taken of me with my breasts smashed together and bulging out of my shirt; these photos are the ones I have chosen to put in my baby's scrapbook.

While I knew that I would appreciate the results of my natural breast-enhancement plan, I had given little thought to the fact that a by-product of my plan was my own personal built-in fan club. My sweet baby girl loves my breasts more tenderly and exuberantly than any lover (or fondler) ever has. Even with her occasional bites and "oh-crap-I-should-really-trim-the-baby's-nails" pinches, she is more devoted to, and enamored of my breasts than anyone else has ever been. I mean, she wakes me in the middle of the night just because she wants to check on them and make sure they are still there and intact. She pulls down my shirt in public just because she misses them so. Recently, I spent fifteen minutes in a conversation with friends with one breast fully exposed because my delightful daughter, unbeknownst to me, had seen fit to make sure my nipple got more daylight (and my friends had been too "polite" to bring my attention to my semi-nudity).

Of course I love my daughter for many reasons, but the more she loves my breasts, the more I love her. Her uninhibited, pure devotion to my breasts has helped me to love them, too, regardless of their size. Her role in making my boobs what they are, and loving them for it, puts me forever in her debt. How old is too old for breastfeeding? I wish I still had that black mesh bra with the satin trim. I would squeeze my enormous boobs into it just to watch the A cups runneth over. And if my daughter asked for the bra, I would give it to her.

BASKETBALL AND BREASTFEEDING

MANDY COHEN

*T*HURSDAY MORNING—4:15 A.M.—ATLANTA
It's eerily quiet in the deserted hallway on the 24th floor. I knock on the secret door. No answer. I knock a little harder and wait. Nothing. I try one more time. The door finally opens. I sigh in relief as a man hands me a package. "They said you were coming for these."

Yesterday—9:00 a.m.—Phillips Arena
Game day. I work for ESPN. I travel around the country every week producing NBA games. I have done this kind of thing for over twenty years, but this year it's different. This year, I am a mom, a breastfeeding mom. As you can probably guess, I work mostly with men.

This morning, I arrive at our TV truck and go immediately to our operations manager, Greg. Usually my first questions involve set up and interview rooms, but these days I need to know one thing, "Where can I pump?" Want to make a man blush? Ask this question.

Greg frowns at me behind his rosy cheeks and I know it's not going to be pretty. "Follow me," he says.

We arrive at a small storeroom with no lock on the door and a window facing a busy hallway. I look over at him and laugh. "It's the best I could do. Sorry," he says.

I shrug my shoulders. I've done worse. NBA arenas are not set up for pumping. I have pumped in a corner with someone holding a curtain up, in a bathroom stall, in the mascot's locker

31

room, at the first aide station, in a parked car, in the audio room, you name it. So this small storeroom is actually not so bad. I thank him and head into practice.

Our interview goes long. I'm overdue for a pump and about to burst. "Who wants to go straight to lunch, I'm starving!" Jon, my analyst, says as I herd everyone toward the car.

I explain that I have to stop at the hotel and when he asks why, I answer, "Because if I don't go pump right this minute, you'll all be having breast milk for lunch." It's not easy to embarrass ex-NBA players, but there stand three men with three identical blushes.

When we arrive at the hotel, I rush off, telling the guys I'll meet them at the restaurant. I run up to my room, pump out eight ounces, put them in the small fridge and hurry back down for our production meeting. After an hour of basketball talk, I change into my game time clothes. Thank goodness maternity wear has entered the work force. I grab a nursing dress that passes for a simple black dress but will come apart easily, making it much more efficient when I have to race into the storeroom to take care of business later.

With my discrete pump backpack slung on my shoulder, I meet the director downstairs and we head back over to the arena for the game. It's 3:00 p.m. Two more pumping sessions on deck before tip off. I've gotten used to structuring my entire day around pump times. I've had to rearrange everything to accommodate, but the crew I work with is wonderful. We do coaches meetings earlier, we rehearse later, and no one seems to mind. At 4:00, I grab my cell and my pump and tell the assistant director I'll be indisposed for a while but text me if you need anything.

The storeroom is dark as I enter. I plop myself down on the floor under the window, hoping no one can see in. I hook myself up and begin answering emails. The doorknob rattles. I look up helplessly. There is no quick way to cover up so I stand my ground. The door opens. The trainer stands there, staring at me. "Hi," I say.

Stuttering, he reaches for a stack of towels. "Uh, I just, uh, need some…"

I smile at him. He is so rattled he forgets the towels and backs out of the room. I pick up my cell and text the truck: Can you send the runner to the storeroom please?

Two minutes later our female runner knocks on the door. "Did you need something?" I yell out to her, "I'm sorry to ask this, but can you just stand guard for me?"

She laughs and says, "No problem."

Twenty minutes later, I'm done, ten ounces in the bag and it's back to work. I drop the milk into a cooler full of ice saved just for me.

Coaches meetings, dinner, rehearsals and some transmission problems and suddenly it's 7:00 p.m., only a half hour to air. I jump up, grab my backpack and look at the director. He smiles and says, "Going to get pumped up for the game?" He says this to me every night. He's a dad and he gets it. "I'll hold down the fort while you're gone." I grab the runner and race back to the storeroom. I won't be able to do the full pump but if I don't do at least fifteen minutes, I won't make it through the game. No one tries to enter the room this time, and I make it back to the truck with five minutes to spare.

The first half goes by in a flash. Atlanta is up five. My boobs are already beginning to hurt but I know I'll have to stick it out until the game is over. With ten seconds left, Denver ties it up. We're going to overtime. I whimper but know there is nothing I can do except pray I don't start leaking. The game finally ends and we go off the air.

The guys and I pile into an SUV for the ride back to the hotel. I get in the back and announce to everyone, "You aren't going to like this, but if I don't pump immediately, I might pass out from the pain." No one says anything but I can almost hear the blushing. I don't care. I whip out my cover, drape it over my dress and start. All you can hear in the car is the whoosh,

whoosh, whoosh of the pump and my loud sigh as the pressure lessens. With traffic, it's a twenty-minute ride back to the hotel, just enough time. As we pull up to the lobby, I say, "Anyone up for a drink?" They all mumble yes as they scramble away from the car. I run up to my room, transfer the day's milk into the fridge and meet everyone at the bar. I have a water and hang for an hour, working off the adrenaline from the day. Then it's back upstairs to pump once more before bed. It's midnight. I have a 6:00 a.m. flight. I set the alarm for 3:45 a.m. and try and close my eyes for a few hours.

As the alarm blares, I roll, bleary-eyed, out of bed and grab the pump. One quick session before I head to the airport. I pack all the bags of milk from the fridge in two small travel coolers. But I need my ice packs. They are at the concierge on the 24th floor. Most hotels will freeze the bags for me but I have to retrieve them in the morning before I go. Thus here I am at 4:15 a.m., knocking on the secret employee door, praying someone answers.

Now that I have my precious ice packs, I add them to the coolers and head to the airport. Security is always an adventure. Sometimes, I breeze right through no questions asked. Sometimes, I have to defend the rights of all breastfeeding mothers worldwide and scream and yell until they let me through with my "liquid gold." There isn't a person in the universe that can make me pour out, leave behind, or check my bags of milk. This morning is a level-five on the annoyance meter.

The pump goes through the x-ray machine. I love watching the TSA guy's face. A frown and a yell, "BAG CHECK!"

I lean over and say, "It's just my breast pump." His face turns that lovely shade of pink so familiar to me. They take my pump and open it up. They have no idea what they are looking at and clearly just want it over with. They shove it back at me, completely ignoring the 70 ounces of liquid I'm carrying and is currently coming out the conveyor belt. I smile sweetly as I repack the pump, gather up my milk and my bags, and set out for the gate. Five hours until I'm home again.

On board, I stow my carry on and put the pump under the seat in front of me. After all, I'm going to need it shortly. Two hours into the flight I have the enviable task of pumping in the very roomy (not!) airplane bathroom. I'm happily pumping away when the lock slides from the outside. Yet again, no time to cover up so the flight attendant gets an eyeful when he throws open the door. "OH! I'm so sorry! I didn't ... You should have ... Oh God." And the door slams closed. I've been walked in on so many times, I have not only lost count but figure I left my dignity back at Madison Square Garden months ago. And I don't care. I'm bringing home 80 ounces of boob juice. I rock!

Thursday —8:43 a.m.—Los Angeles

We touch down at LAX. I gather my things and scramble off the plane. I've been gone 40 hours but it feels like a week. A taxi whisks me home. My husband comes out to greet me, holding our daughter. I snuggle her to my chest while simultaneously undoing my nursing bra. She is on the boob before I even make it through the door. I think the cabbie might have seen nipple. Oh well, add him to the list.

Final tally on this trip: Times walked in on—two; Security issues —one; Awkward moments—nine; Blushes induced—12. Not too bad. And lucky me, I get to do it all again next week. Bring it on!

THE SHIELD

AMANDA ROSEN-PRINZ

THE SHIELD. The *fucking* shield. Before giving birth to my son, I hardly even knew what a nipple shield was, let alone why one might be necessary during breastfeeding. In fact, I never gave much thought to breastfeeding at all while I was pregnant. I took for granted that it was just something I would do. My mother breastfed me and my mother-in-law breastfed my husband; of course I would breastfeed my children as well.

During my pregnancy I focused my energy and anxiety on ensuring the perfect, natural birth experience. I took extensive and comprehensive birthing classes and practiced relaxation and deep abdominal breathing. I did prenatal yoga, bodywork and acupuncture to ready my body for birth. I gave little thought to what would come after the big day. Never mind the whole child-rearing and parenting thing—what about sustaining life through breastmilk? That's not a tall order or anything. In the end, I did get my "perfect" birth experience after all. But oh the hubris! I should have known that a gal can't have it all so easily.

After a lovely and uneventful birth, my healthy and beautiful baby boy was placed on my chest in order to benefit from prized skin-to-skin bonding time. It would also be an opportunity for him to enjoy his first meal at the milk buffet. Unfortunately, he had a bit of trouble latching. I told myself that he just spent 20 hours working his way out of my womb, so I should give him a break and we will keep trying. I tried not to stress, but things only got worse.

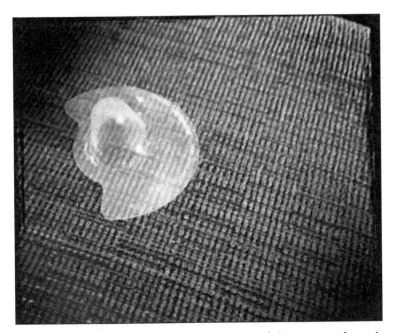

Latching was a battle, and it was painful. Hours of work and tears produced only minutes of actual nursing. Luz, the hospital lactation consultant, offered helpful suggestions. "Feed him the sandwich, Mommy," she jovially instructed while excruciatingly squeezing my breasts into a rough approximation of a sandwich. My son must not have been in the mood for a booby Big Mac just yet because he declined that offer as well.

My nipples were diagnosed by the hospital nurses as flat. One nurse brought me ice cubes in the middle of the night to chill my nipples into submission, and bring them out into more erect, latchable forms. Another offered sugar water, presumably to con the baby into thinking he was just having a little dessert. Meanwhile, my ample breasts became even more plentiful as they painfully engorged and swallowed up my supposedly flat nipples.

The nurses offered bottles and formula but I was hip to that. When I refused, they next prescribed a little silicone disk with a pointy cone-like bump in the middle. It looked like a clear miniature version of a wicked witch's hat. A nipple shield. It worked like an oversized artificial nipple to help the baby latch—breastfeeding training wheels, if you will. I sought guidance from the Internet where a virtual cornucopia of horror stories terrified me: The baby will become addicted to the shield and never again accept your breast! The shield is not a panacea and might confuse the baby's latch even more! It could affect milk production! It may lead to plugged ducts and mastitis! He might grow a third eye! It seemed that the shield was in fact as wicked as its appearance would suggest. I was duly warned. I politely declined the nipple shield but took it home with me along with all the other free hospital loot like extra mesh panties and dinosaur-sized mega-maxi pads.

The good news was that I was making a sufficient amount of milk, so I began pumping right away and looked for any method to get my baby to consume my hearty milk. We tried a tiny spoon (too messy, but adorable), a syringe (too time consuming, and mildly creepy) and, once I gave in and got over my fear of nipple confusion, finally a bottle (just right, but shameful, as if admitting defeat).

My baby was thriving on his pumped milk but still refused what I once believed were my glorious nipples (at least all the other men in my life thus far had viewed them as such). I met with a well-intended lactation consultant who ultimately, after collecting her fee, kindly shrugged their shoulders. Were we not meant to be in a successful breastfeeding relationship? His high arched palate and my semi-flat nipples seemed to be an incompatible match. Nevertheless, we kept trying.

Complicating matters, my baby cried all the time for no discernible reason. The pediatrician diagnosed him with *colic*, which is a disorder characterized by a baby crying all the time *for no discernible reason*. And there is no cure for colic. Needless to say, it was difficult to work with him when he was so easily frustrated. He cried. I cried. After two weeks of this insanity, I finally pulled out the hospital-provided nipple shield and rinsed it off. I reluctantly applied it to my nipple like using a condom for the first time, and nervously put my son to the breast. Angels sang as he effortlessly latched on and gulp, gulp, gulped down my milk. He was no longer crying, my breasts were no longer red and hard, and we were both sated. However, I was resolute that this was only a temporary solution. I called back the lactation consultant and she confirmed that he was getting enough milk through the shield. Now that I was sure he was actually being nourished, we made a plan that I would continue to work at weaning him from the shield. This entailed using the shield to initiate a latch and then stealthily yanking it away without the baby noticing as he continued to nurse on my bare nipple. This did not work. I am not suggesting that my son was a genius baby, but he was not fooled by those shenanigans.

Every time I attempted to remove the shield and shove my naked nipple into his adorable little mouth he didn't have a clue what to do with it. He smiled or giggled in my face, as if he was onto the sly trick I was trying to play on him. "What is this nonsense?" he asked me with his pure blue eyes and furrowed brow. His humor provided a very limited window before the screaming commenced and out came the nipple shield to the rescue, while I sing-songed apologies for offending his baby sense of decency.

Days turned into weeks, which turned into months, and we were still going strong with that shield. It was official, my son had developed a silicone fetish. He was in love with a pretend nipple when he had the real thing right there in front of him. Would he grow up to be into bondage and kinky sex? The months trudged on and his love affair with the shield continued to blossom as my delusions about weaning him from it were swept away. Here I was, this brand new mama who had once been petrified of letting anything not organic or considered "natural" touch any part of my baby's body, now regularly offering him a piece of synthetic material to suck on all day (and night) long. He preferred the emotionless rubbery slickness of the shield to my *au-natural* bosom.

I carried the nipple shield in my bra like a talisman. I couldn't go anywhere without it, lest my son need to eat or find comfort at any given moment. I had fantasized about being one of those mothers who proudly and cavalierly whipped her boob out whenever and wherever. Instead, I had to consider the sanitation and whereabouts of my nipple shield at all times. "Just spit on it and wipe it off," suggested one well-seasoned lactation consultant at a breastfeeding support group. I couldn't quite bring myself to be that blasé, but over time I became more lax about whether the shield was properly sterilized between uses. After all, this baby was noshing twelve or more times a day! I became complacent about the shield being coated with boob sweat and sprinkled with dried milk from the previous feeding. Anyhow, that's how my son liked it best, with a little old milk residue aging like a fine stinky cheese and a nice coating of aromatic mommy juice.

The shield became my son's lovey. As he grew older he would engage in his own version of foreplay with it, letting it tickle his face and jiggling it around in his hand like a rattle before getting down with the main course. Meanwhile, I felt embarrassed and dejected about breastfeeding. I was too timid to nurse openly with the shield because I believed it would betray my secret motherly failing. Many people who knew my dirty little secret commended me on my achievement and fortitude in the face of breastfeeding adversity. Some expressed that I might have broken a special world record by nursing so long with a shield as we approached the two year mark, my son merrily nursing away with his faux nipple fetish in full swing. I knew I should feel proud of my breastfeeding achievement but I couldn't help but feel sad about the barrier between my son and me.

And so it went; for nearly two years I used a nipple shield to feed my son. He never figured out how to feed from my un-shielded breast. Today the nipple shield is a faded memory for my son as he nears his third birthday. With the recent birth of my second child (who incidentally nurses just fine, go figure!) my son became curious about his own nursing story. Watching his mommy with her breasts hanging out all day naturally got him asking some questions. "WHATCHAREYOUDOING Mommy?" he asked me one day. "I'm feeding your baby sister with milk from my breasts," I replied proudly. I sometimes ask him if he recalls his old friend the nipple shield. He tells me that he remembers, but I am not so convinced, as he often follows up by asking me if I remember that he is a Tyrannosaurus Rex, "RAWR!" The preschooler's brain is a tough nut to crack.

It is now clear to me that this experience, which I spent two years obsessing over as my tragic inadequacy as a woman, was just a fleeting moment for my son but a defining moment for me as a mother. As with most things in parenting, we do the best we can and while we may worry that we are damaging our children beyond repair, it often turns out that they don't know any better and love us just the same. While my son is none the wiser about our tumultuous breastfeeding relationship, it remains a bittersweet journey for me.

The shield. The *fucking* nipple shield, as I semi-affectionately called it. Even though it established a barrier between my son and me, it was the very thing that saved our breastfeeding relationship.

CABBAGE-WRAPPED BREASTS, ANYONE?

HELEN TAN

ABBAGE-WRAPPED BREASTS—sounds like an inviting dish, doesn't it? The origin of this "family recipe" dates back to 1993, the year my eldest child was born.

During my first pregnancy, my husband and I devoured books on pregnancy and baby care like voracious termites. Breastfeeding became a common topic of discussion.

"It says here the colostrum in breast milk is important for a baby's development. It's recommended that you breastfeed for at least the first two weeks." From his gleaming smile, it was obvious my husband thought this was a fantastic idea.

Of course, why wouldn't he? After all, he wasn't the one with the breasts. He wasn't the one who would have to wake up several times throughout the night and tend to a starving, screaming baby.

But in all fairness, I had to agree with him when the books reiterated how breastfeeding would boost the baby's immune system. For two accounts-trained professionals, breastfeeding seemed the only way to go. Dollar signs scrolled through our minds as we projected mega-savings on milk powder and medical bills.

Well, the delivery day came and it was time to put all our knowledge skimmed from books into practice. Breastfeeding didn't look as though it would pose any problems. After all, what could be more difficult than squirming, screaming, suffering through labour pain?

Soon after delivery, a senior nurse came into my hospital

room and asked, "Are you opting for total breastfeeding, partial, or milk powder?"

"Total breastfeeding." I beamed with confidence.

My husband beamed with pride. All looked set for a blissful bonding between my baby and me. That was until my baby howled and the nurse wheeled him into my room.

"Wipe your breasts clean and I'll hand you the baby."

I propped myself into position, followed the nurse's instruction and waited for the all-important handover. I waited to showcase my well-fed knowledge, and therefore expected skills, in breastfeeding. The nurse placed a struggling, hungry and still-howling baby into my arms.

"Let him latch onto your nipple. Why can't you do it? Oh, I see the problem. Your right nipple is too short. Pull it out!"

Problem? Huh, what? All my panic buttons burst. Sirens sounded in my mind. The word "FAILURE" in capital letters weighed down on me and squeezed all confidence from my system.

The nurse tugged and pinched my nipple. I bit my lips, cowered in silence as she manhandled my nipple like a potter moulding a clay sculpture. Finally, she managed to educate me as to the finer points of breastfeeding. My baby latched onto my "pulled out" nipple but there was no milk.

"Not to worry," the nurse said. "The milk will usually come by the third day." She instructed me to continue and allow my baby to suckle so as to stimulate milk production.

On the third day, we were discharged from the hospital and it was "home, sweet home."

We bustled around our apartment, arranging the cot, changing diapers, and of course, snapping pictures of our "little darling." My breasts hardened. Darting pain shot through them. Too immersed in my newly discovered "goo-goo ga-ga" euphoria, I ignored the swelling and pain.

By the time the pain became too acute for me to bear, it was too late. I tried a hot sponge, but those two concrete masses felt reinforced with cast iron. I tried feeding my baby, but he couldn't latch on. His hunger, his struggle, his screaming escalated my pain and panic.

I gulped down my pride, prepared a bottle of milk and popped it into the baby's searching mouth. Then I thrust the baby into my husband's arms. I had more urgent matters to tend to.

"Look, Dar, look at my breasts. They're so hard. It's soooo painful. What should I doooo? Aargh, pain..." I bared my breasts, Clark Kent-style, but instead of showing a Super "S" logo, my action exposed solid rock formations.

"Oh my God, what are those? Gross, you look like Arnold Schwarzenegger! Look at those veins. I don't know, call Dr. Lim, he's the specialist."

I did exactly that, I rang my gynecologist. "May I speak to Dr. Lim PLEASE?"

"Dr. Lim isn't available. He's at the hospital. Maybe I can help you?"

"My breasts are engorged. They're so hard, so heavy, so painful. Can Dr. Lim give me a pill? I want to stop breastfeeding."

"Aiyah, for this type of minor matter, you don't need Dr. Lim's help. Just get some cabbage leaves, the ones with very thick veins. Put them in the fridge until you need to use them. When your breasts become engorged, wrap a cold leaf around each breast. Find the tightest bra you have and strap the leaves in."

"Huh, are you sure this will work? It's very painful you know. There's so much milk jammed in my breasts. They feel like lumps of hardened cheese."

"You're lucky you have milk. Some people don't even have a single drop of milk when they want it. The Singapore Association for Breastfeeding is *dying* for donation."

"Ask them to send their container trucks over NOW!"

"You're so funny. Go, go and try the cabbage leaves." With that, the nurse ended our conversation.

I doubted her words, thinking she just wanted me and my whines off the line. But I was desperate. If someone had asked me to paint my breasts blue as a cure, I would have done so. Maybe using cabbage leaves was not such a bad option.

I sent my husband out in search of the cabbage with the thickest veins. He bought a monstrous cabbage with awesome veins, which I promptly stored in the fridge. As soon as it was cold enough, I followed the nurse's instructions. I strapped those leaves onto my concrete breasts with the tightest bra I could find.

Surprise—such a great relief and release! My breasts, massaged by those wondrous veins, softened to their natural state. The milk started to flow. I cleaned my breasts, fed a satisfied baby and floated with the adrenaline of a successful breastfeeding mum. Aaah ... the pleasure those cabbage leaves gave me was beyond expression.

My husband thought it a waste to throw the leaves away. They looked limp but surely they were still edible. But in case anyone is wondering, cabbage leaves stewed in milk has *never* been served as a dish in our family.

I have shared this cabbage recipe with several friends and the verdict is unanimous: nothing beats it.

That's all folks, it's a wrap!

(INTO AND) OUT OF THE MOUTHS OF BABES

JESSICA CLAIRE HANEY

I *TRY TO RESIST THE PULL to fulfill his desires. He craves my attention, my embrace, my gaze, but I want the moment to be mine alone. I am successful only until he says my name. Then my will is gone, and I'm his.*
"Jessica! Jess!"

When my son was two, he took to yelling out my first name when a few rounds of "Mommy" hadn't yielded desirable results. He usually employed this strategy to get my attention when I was cooking or typing—when my back was turned or my forehead wrinkles betrayed the fact that his activity at that moment was not the first thing on my mind. With his eyebrows arched in gleeful discovery and his chubby index finger pointing to his newest project, excitement was the dominant undertone in his voice. Still, there was an insistence that registered to my ears as more demanding than anything. Feeling guilty for multitasking my motherhood, I usually gave in.

Being on a first-name basis with my son made me feel like I was both his equal and his servant—a familiar dynamic. Since the beginning of our relationship, he and I had spent a lot of time breastfeeding. At two, my son's love affair with my breasts still sizzled. The concept of my body as both mine and the boy's had long been a challenge for my husband, even before the boy was walking or talking. Or calling out my first name.

His language and cognition had matured by the time he was two, but his desire for my body blurred boundaries, challenging

46

me. It was one thing to be felt up when he was an incoherent blob. But it felt different when he could say to me, "I wanna nurse you, Mommy" and "other side" while trying to wedge his whole arm under my bra and creep his fingers toward my unoccupied nipple, as though this time I might decide I like it instead of telling him, "Move your hand." I began instinctively to hug my chest, pressing my unsupporting arm against the dormant breast, sometimes cupping myself, or pulling him off to stop the groping.

Nursing used to be the panacea for all ills: hunger, fear, fatigue. By age two, we were on a more predictable schedule, but my son's eyes would still flash when I got naked like lollipops were taped to my chest. He'd pretend to reach out and coyly tell me he wanted to nurse, just because he could say the words, and then would proceed to ponder my genitalia, fascinated with the embouchure required to say "vagina." His mouth played with different tones and tempos for the word. I both laughed and cringed when he began toggling between the V-word and "Jessica," whispering as though both three-syllable words were magical mantras holding the key to a delicious mystery. Perhaps they are.

Fortunately, though, when we had a real "conversation," my toddler son usually displayed an uncanny situational appropriateness, using my first name only in a way he might have heard from his father. I always hoped this meant that as long as we continued to breastfeed, I would be safe from hearing, "I wanna nurse you, Jess."

But I also didn't factor in to what extent he would soak up— and repeat as his own—phrases I'd say. After I'd reluctantly nursed him once or twice after exercising and apparently made some comment about the taste of sweat, he got the connection. One day, a few months before he turned three, he turned up to look at me from the jogging stroller and asked, "Are your nipples a little salty?"

At any other time in my life, I'd have assumed this was a

line from a porn flick featuring an aerobics instructor. But it was my son. Talking about *me*.

From everything I read and thought about, it seemed like my son might be ready to wean. And I was ready to have my body back and no longer a subject of interest to my son's palate. So I casually suggested in the car one day, looking back at him in the rearview mirror, "You know, I was thinking you might be ready to be done nursing when you turn three." He didn't say much, and I mentioned it maybe just one other time.

But then we went to a farm and came across piglets that were just three days old. I asked him, on video, to talk about what the piggies were doing. I have pixelized documentation of him saying, "They're nursing! I like nursing! And I'm going to stop nursing when it's my birthday!"

Truer words were never spoken.

Note: *Portions of this essay were previously published at the blog for* Motherverse Magazine, *which is no longer in publication.*

JUNGLE JUICE

ELIANA OSBORN

IT'S SO WET I CAN'T SMELL the sulfur of the volcano, even though it is right ahead of me. Instead, it appears we've been hiking for a mile down a gravel path, rainy season in full force, just to read about geological happenings. My four-year-old is a blueberry in his insulated raincoat, hood pulled tight. Strapped to my front in the baby carrier, Owen is six months old and having the time of his life. He's got a hat and a waterproofed nursing cover draped around him. I've got my purple North Face jacket open to shield his arms and an umbrella overhead.

As we stand at the edge of the abyss, all I see are clouds. Every so often, though, the fog lifts and a crater appears, striated with color and puffing little bursts of steam up to join the clouds all around.

"Should we try the jungle path for another view?" My husband can tell this isn't the Costa Rican vacation I thought we were getting into. We're here, though, so what else is there to do but hike.

It's our second day in Central America and we've ventured out of San Jose to Volcan Poas for a little nature. The best part of traveling with an infant? Everyone wants to touch the fat little white baby. We even got to skip the line at customs when he was hysterical—can't imagine that happening in the U.S.

The boys run ahead, hoping to spot tapirs or spider monkeys in the jungle, while I trudge along with my awkward front load. It is quiet under the canopy of huge leaves protecting me from the rain, only isolated drips and bird sounds. Baby Owen starts to fuss and I realize he's hungry.

Sitting on my rain coat, I take off the baby carrier. I'm sweating in the steamy weather and so is the baby. We lose the layers and I try to angle his hat to cover his face from stray drops plopping on his nose. I hook him up. He's eating away, thrilled at the fresh air and milk. I'm crouched a bit awkwardly, watching a line of carpenter ants carry leaf pieces double their size. My butt's a bit damp, the light's a bit dim, and the side of my breast is getting a nice cool breeze.

This is how it is to be a mom for much of the world, taking care of your child's needs outside. No hidden nursing lounge, no rear-facing booth at a restaurant. Part of the natural world, not separate from it. We take our time, Owen and I.

The zen moment passes. It is semi-dark. I'm alone in the middle of nowhere. I have a baby and I'm wet. So very wet. The baby carrier is hot and wet, and neither Owen nor I is excited to wriggle back in. But we do it. Owen's topped off for a while, full enough, but I know it won't last long. It is hard to eat much when you're a desert baby in the middle of a rain forest.

Photos from our trip are a sequence of me looking awkward with a baby growing off my chest, a ripple of fat at my waist and an annoyed look on my face. Look, Eliana's nursing on a beach with spider monkeys trying to steal the backpack. Look, Eliana's nursing on a suspension bridge, trying to walk and feed to keep up with the hiking group. Eliana's nursing on a restaurant porch, trying to eat tender sea bass left-handed so it won't fall in her lap. Ah, the magic.

HANGIN' OUT

AMA CHRISTABEL NSIAH-BUADI

MY BOOBS DON'T BELONG TO ME. For now. They're on loan to my daughter, and that's really okay. This discovery created an existential crisis in me for a little while—"Have my breasts ever really belonged to me? Will they ever belong to me long after I stop breastfeeding? How close to my knees will they be once everything is said and done?"—but for now, I'm kinda over it. I think. In the final analysis, the decision about when the "girls" would have to come out on display stopped being mine the moment I vowed to stick with breastfeeding.

And while my decision to continue breastfeeding (despite the challenges of blocked ducts and mastitis) was a profound moment that involved tears and lots of hugs, the realization that "my boobs no longer belong to me" was quite the opposite, which is crazy, given that the particular moment happened in downtown Los Angeles. As in LaLa Land, the place where dreams go to die. Picture this: I'm waiting to be interviewed about the challenges of breastfeeding for the local public radio station, when I get a call from the journalist (who is also a friend, for full disclosure), who can't find a place to park.

The thing is, we're both on a deadline: she has to be back in her office in fifteen minutes, while my four-month-old daughter, whom I'll call "Aretha Carey," because she has the lung power of Aretha Franklin and the vocal range of Mariah Carey, is letting me know that she is getting really, really hungry and will run out of patience in about ... fifteen minutes.

We both had to make this happen. And fast. So I steeled myself. "Get ready," I told myself. "The girls are going to make their first major prime-time appearance today."

My journo-friend pulled up at Seventh and Figueroa, which is always bustling with foot traffic from construction workers, tourists, and locals. It doesn't smell particularly great, either.

"Do you mind doing the interview in the car?" she asked me.

"Uh shhhuuuuuuuree, we can do that...?" I said. I agreed because I trust her. She's a mother of two herself, and I know she's completely sympathetic to my feelings, which right now include slight reluctance.

"There's another thing. I'm going to have to keep my eye out, because we probably shouldn't be parked here, but I can't find anywhere else."

I started laughing before she even finishes her sentence. I got it: after all, I'm a journalist myself. When you're on deadline, you have to make it work, no matter where you are. Plus, she just wanted to ask me a few questions. The journalist in me was excited about helping her get her story. I hadn't had to deal with this type of work pressure in a while! I started to weigh things up: three questions ... twelve minutes ... maybe fifteen... Before I could complete my thought, she said, "Hey, and if you need to, you can just feed babygirl in the car...."

"In the WHAT? Where? Here, in front of all of these possibly crazy people?" I thought to myself. Which is why I asked her in a very calm tone, "But what if she starts fussing while we're talking?"

"That's totally fine, it'll be relevant to the piece! It'll be 'sweet'!"

Hmm, sweet indeed. Someone was about to get a free peep show, and I wasn't down with that at all. Complaints aside, I was in awe, really. Her creativity was awesome, and I absolutely trusted her, in spite of my concerns.

My modesty fought back for a second, though. I surveyed the area to see who my potential audience was. There were some construction workers (all men), another man pushing his belongings in a trolley, who seemed quite intrigued by the "two ladies and a baby in a car with a microphone" situation developing, a few lost tourists and the lunch crowd ... oh, and the people in traffic. Oh good, so not many people, I grumbled quietly to myself.

I took a deep breath. "Okaylet'sdothis." We jumped in the car. Babygirl started fussing. I looked at my journo-friend. The "girls" came out. My daughter looked at me as if to say, "That's right, now let's get to business." So, we did. She started eating and my journo-friend started asking questions.

"So you've written about some of the challenges you faced when you started breastfeeding. Can you tell me about that?"

The irony of the situation wasn't lost on me. Talking about breastfeeding challenges while nervously popping the "girls" out—in public—to feed my baby. I looked to my right, and I swear I saw one of the construction workers slow down. I stared him down as my daughter searched for the nipple she'd let go of just seconds earlier.

I started to rattle my answer off, trying to sound as focused as possible. I was convinced I sounded like an idiot. Externally I was all smiles, happy to share my revelations with this journalist, and then,

Glug ... glug ... glug...

Babygirl was enjoying her lunch and letting us know. Hmm. what to do? Ignore the sound, or acknowledge it? What does a broadcast professional do in this situation? I decided to acknowledge it: "...and even as I'm talking to you, I'm feeding my daughter in the middle of downtown Los Angeles, ah-hahahaha!"

I sounded like a prat. My journo-friend was kind. She moved on to the next set of questions and I answered them, paying no attention to the crowd we may or may not have had. Then I noticed the journalist looking away from me. Clearly my answers weren't that interesting. "Is everything okay?" I asked.

She nodded, but quickly added, "They're towing the car behind us. I'm sorry, really I am listening to you, but we're gonna have to go..."

The hustler in me kicked into gear. Out came the nipple (Babygirl was sated, at least for now, so I figured I had bought myself thirty minutes), and the "girls" went back in. Then, out of nowhere, I blurted, "Tell them that you have a nursing mother in here; tell them that my baby was hungry and she needed to eat and that we had to stop to feed her! I'll keep feeding her to make the point if I have to!"

I sounded indignant. I caught myself and laughed. I'd gone from worrying about the world seeing my boobs, to being prepared to breastfeed in public to help a friend avoid a parking ticket.

Was what I suggested a little manipulative? Maybe. But in that moment, I realized that I'd finally embraced my new identity as a mother and that felt powerful and liberating.

PRETTY

LACY LYNN

I ASKED MY DAUGHTER TO UNDRESS for our shower as I did the same. I leaned over the tub, turned on the faucet and dangled my fingers through the running water, waiting for just the right temperature. I glanced to my side just in time to see my half-dressed daughter swing her leg over the tub, eager to play in the water. I kindly said, "Deary, you must finish undressing first or you're gonna get your clothes all wet." Once I saw her start to remove the rest of her clothing I took my attention back to the water. Then I hear, "Poo-eety!"

I hear this word a thousand times a day. Pretty snow. Pretty butterflies. Pretty rainbow. Pretty hair. Pretty dress. It's now routine to reply with a universal, "Yes, it is very pretty." But my quick-fire acknowledgement wasn't enough on this occasion. She further insisted, "Poo-eety! Poo-eety!" Then I felt a slight tug at my nipple. A bit confused I looked away from the water and at the source of the tug. It was, of course, my daughter. "Poo-eety mama! Poo-eety booooooob."

I have never once, that I can recall, used a word such as this to describe my breasts in front of my daughter. I've often referred to my breasts as food for her, as in when I ask, "Do you want a booby snack?" while motioning the sign for breastfeed, or saying "It's time to snuggle" for times when I wanted to be less obvious in front of others. Most certainly have I never used a phrase like, "Look, deary. Mama has pretty boobs." I glanced at my breasts intently and for a moment became lost in thought trying to match the word "pretty" with what looked to me to be nothing more than goat teats.

Before becoming pregnant I had a pair of beautiful C-cups that leaned over a bar nicely and, I'm certain, played a part in attracting my daughter's father. When I became pregnant they turned into voluptuous D-cups. Man, did I love those hormone-enraged breasts! I had never felt sexier or more beautiful than when I had those things on me. When my milk came in 20 hours after the birth of my daughter, they became udders. The milk-filled veins throbbed across my breasts just the same as when the cows came down from the fields to our barn ready to be milked, their engorged bags squirting the aisle full of milk all the way to their stanchions. I was a cow, and that made me feel ugly.

But I was one proud cow for sure. I provided every delicious drop of milk my daughter ever needed as well as donated gallons to my milk babies (babies who receive donated breastmilk either through a milk bank or through a local milk-sharing network). For the length of time I breastfed, I associated lots of words with my breasts.

Engorged berthas
Squirters
Mother leakers
Mega mastitis ouchers
Nipple crackies
Milk machines
Rock hard mamas

...and as time passed and weaning started, they sadly became known as...

Floppy boppies.

Nothing came close to "pretty" in my mind. What could my daughter possibly be thinking? My daughter will be turning two years old tomorrow, and it's been three months since we last nursed. My once-glorious milk makers are now meager A-cups. Sure, my breasts have been plenty purposeful, but pretty?

"Poo-eety mama."

I looked past my dangling, floppy boobs, and there stood my daughter, staring straight into my eyes with a precious smile on her face and gently tugging away yet.

"What did you say?" I asked, still in disbelief.

"Mama! Boooooooob! Poo-eeeety!" Then she looked down at herself, pointed at her own chest and said, "Pretty!"

I looked at my little daughter and laughed to myself. Although I recognized long ago how beautiful nursing is, I had unknowingly created a base for a healthy self-image for my daughter, to become secure in her own beauty in this too-often harsh world.

I kissed the bundle of blonde curls atop her head and replied, "Yes, my deary. Pretty! Thank you for reminding me of something I've long forgotten." I was one proud retired cow.

ABUNDANCE IS OVERRATED

KARI O'DRISCOLL

I TOOK THE CLASSES. I dragged my husband along to each and every one. We saw the gruesome birth videos. (Well, I saw them. I'm pretty sure he turned his head in fear and disgust and whistled a jaunty tune until they were over.) We learned to diaper a newborn, listened to the pros and cons of disposable versus cloth, epidural versus "natural birth," midwives and home births versus traditional hospital births. We were told that breastfeeding is best but that it isn't always easy or convenient, and that pacifiers are fraught with perils for baby tooth development and that you should never ever put your baby down with a bottle by themselves or allow them to sleep on their stomachs until they can roll over.

We made smug choices while our little peanut was still nestled safely inside: no binkies, breastfeeding only, no co-sleeping, and cloth diapers. I would try my best to do a natural birth in the hospital but if it became too much, I would opt for an epidural. Forget the torturous-sounding perineal stretches to prevent tearing—that's what catgut is for. I'd rather have stitches afterward than ask my poor squeamish husband to knead my vagina like so much pizza dough and risk it never bouncing back into shape.

For the sake of full disclosure, I'll tell you that the only ideal we managed to stick to was cloth diapers. Thanks to my refusal to pre-stretch and my baby's desire to come out rotated posteriorly, her forehead wedged firmly up against my tailbone, I ended up getting an inordinate number of stitches in my hoo-ha. The baby had to be suctioned out and arrived kicking and screaming—an exact mini-replica of Jane Curtin as an SNL Conehead.

Oh, and breastfeeding. Well, somehow my breasts got the wrong message and went into hyperdrive, convinced that instead of one single solitary seven-pound human infant, I gave birth to an entire litter of starving puppies. Within 24 hours of Erin's birth, I was producing enough milk to feed a small country. Not ever having done this before, it took me a while to realize that this was unusual. Life was about to get hard.

Like any good maternity ward nurse, Carlita was determined to get my newborn to latch on to my breast immediately upon her entrance to the world. Once she was cleaned up and weighed and my OB was firmly ensconced on a stool between my thighs, diligently sewing my nether-regions back together, Carlita swaddled my little girl to within an inch of her life and headed over. She whipped the hospital gown off of my left shoulder, exposing the only part of my body that had yet to be bared to the entire room, took one look at my nipple and clucked her tongue. She lowered the baby a little bit and shook her head. I was appalled. I glanced down out of curiosity and didn't notice anything out of the norm. Yep, that was my left breast, looking pretty much the way it always did.

"Oh, boy! We arrrre gonna have to perrrrk this one up!" she announced in a thick accent. She handed the baby off to my husband who was more than a little bit scared to hold her and before either of us could formulate a sentence inquiring what she meant by that, she reached out with her long, red fingernails and gave me an honest-to-God Purple Nerple.

No shit. She tweaked my nipple so hard it brought tears to my eyes. I sat straight up in bed, completely forgetting that there was a needle in my vajayjay, and yelled, "What the…!"

Carlita cocked her head to one side. I am fairly certain she didn't realize there was a human attached to the nipple she had just pinched.

"Oh, honey. You have a flat nipple. The baby cannot latch to that. She needs something standing up. Like this!" She beamed proudly and gestured to my now angry nipple, shriveled and standing at attention. She waggled her fingers at Sean, gesturing for him to hand over the baby, and shoved Erin's head into my breast. Even though she was less than an hour old, my baby's instincts were spot-on. She arched her little body and pushed back. Carlita took no notice of her indignant wailing, tucked my arm beneath the sweet, warm little bundle and used two hands to force Erin's head to my breast until her little round mouth was so full of nipple she couldn't make a sound.

"Therrre is no milk right now, darrrrrling, but you have to keep her to the brrrrreast everrry hour, okay? If you need help, I'm rrrright outside." She waddled out of the room on her silent, white nurse shoes, quite pleased at her handiwork.

"Don't you dare ever let that woman in here again!" I hissed at Sean. I wasn't entirely sure whether I was more pissed off that she had tweaked my still-throbbing nipple without asking (not that I would have given her permission), or that she had made my new baby cry. I just knew I didn't want her around either of us again. God forbid my right nipple was flat, too, and she came in to manhandle me repeatedly! This whole business of nipple tweaking was definitely something they hadn't covered in the prenatal classes. I made a mental note to complain.

My milk arrived with a vengeance the day after Erin was born, swelling my breasts to epic proportions. The sheer pressure coupled with the natural (flat) shape of my nipples meant that Erin couldn't latch on to eat no matter how hard we tried. I had been given a kit of different things at the hospital and tried the silicone nipple shield and the syringe taped to my nipple that dribbled a little formula into her mouth, but by the end of our first day at home, I was beginning to panic that she wasn't getting any milk at all.

I called my doctor and tearfully admitted that I couldn't seem to figure this nursing thing out. She laughed and suggested we meet with the hospital's lactation consultant. I couldn't get there fast enough.

For his part, Sean couldn't believe that "Lactation Consultant" was an actual profession. "So, wait a minute. Do you mean to tell me that it's possible to have a job where I get to check out hergungous boobs all day long in person and not get called a pig?"

I assured him that male lactation consultants were probably not in high demand for just that reason. Riding high on his newfound knowledge and the fantasies it conjured up, he dismissed me with a flap of his hand.

The lactation consultant we met with praised me for not giving up on breastfeeding. She examined my breasts and determined that there was nothing about them that meant I couldn't nurse Erin, but after a few failed attempts in her presence, she pinpointed the issue.

"Ahh! You have too much milk, sweetie. She's trying to latch on, but the skin is too taut and she can't get ahold of anything."

You think? I felt like I had two over-filled water balloons strapped to my chest. I honestly believed that if someone poked me with a needle, my skin would peel back and milk would flood the room.

"I think we need to pump off a little bit to release some of the tension and then she can latch on." Why hadn't I thought of that? It made perfect sense. But when she dragged out a small suitcase and flipped it open, I was certain I had misunderstood. This thing looked to me like some sort of brain-transplanting machine I once saw in a Looney Tunes episode.

The base was a sturdy blue plastic box about the size of a breadbox with two rubber hoses leading out of the sides. The hoses were each attached to the back of a funnel that screwed onto the top of a bottle. There were three dials on the front and a toggle switch. The dials controlled the amount of suction and, I would soon learn, could be turned up so high that my nipple was sucked straight into the funnel and ended up looking like a plastic drinking straw for five minutes after I turned the damn thing off. The consultant didn't recommend ever using the highest setting. Good to know.

Perhaps the most amazing revelation from that day is that breastmilk doesn't come out of one hole in the center of your nipple like I previously imagined. Instead, it comes out of several holes at once; like a shower head. I saw it clearly, thanks to the transparent funnels. And once I was hooked up to the machine and the suction began, it was possible, at least for me, to turn it off and have my breasts continue shooting—not dripping, shooting—milk out of all of those holes for several minutes before stopping. If there had such a thing as the Breastfeeding Olympics, I am certain I would have won the gold for distance. The sheer volume of milk my body produced led me to superathlete status. Unfortunately, it also meant that the standard-issue breast pads—those little cotton disks you put inside your nursing bra to soak up any errant drips of breast milk that would otherwise soil your bra or clothing—were not nearly sturdy enough for my needs. After weeks of experimenting with layers of three or four of them at a time, progressing to burp cloths and finally cutting Super Absorbent Maxi Pads down to size and shoving them inside my bra, I realized that I might not be able to wear anything but a loose-fitting sweatshirt until Erin was weaned.

For the time being, though, my problem was solved, thanks to the industrial double breast pump I rented from the hospital. I was able to pump off about three ounces of milk on either side before letting Erin nurse. This seemed to be just enough to allow her tiny little mouth to fit on my nipple and begin suck-ing. I finally felt as though I was capable of feeding my child!

But, like they say, be careful what you wish for. What I got is something I like to call the "Field of Dreams Dilemma." The more milk your body expresses, the more it makes. It's an evolutionary trick of supply and demand, like when a huge number of people head down to the corner store to buy Cheetos.

This prompts the store to order more Cheetos so they don't run out. Breast milk production works on the same principle. So even though the milk I was pumping off (three oz. per breast on an average of eight times per day) wasn't being consumed, per se, it was being expressed. As far as my hormones knew, I was using a certain volume of milk every day and it needed to keep making that much milk. Every day. All the time. By pumping before nursing, I had created a vicious cycle that prompted my body to make more milk, which resulted in my breasts becoming engorged again, which meant I had to keep pumping it off before Erin could latch on, and so on and so forth for eternity. Or that's what it felt like to me.

The issue of what to do with all of this milk I pumped off remained as well. I was loathe to simply pour it down the drain for several reasons. As a child, I was taught by my frugal parents that waste is one of the paramount sins of mankind and I learned that lesson well. To this day I repurpose the chicken carcass from my store-bought rotisserie chickens, toss it in a pot of water with carrot peelings, old saggy celery and other herbs and veggies that probably ought to be in the compost bin, and make my own chicken stock. Besides, as a new mother, I was still under the starry-eyed impression that one day soon I would enjoy a day out with my girlfriends and I'd need Sean to feed the baby some milk without having to leave my breasts behind. Enter the freezer bag. I was told that frozen breast milk will keep for several months, so I sent Sean back to Babies "R" Us for a box of handy little breast milk freezer bags and filled a couple up every time I pumped. Eight times a day, give or take.

Yeah. Within two weeks my freezer was full of breastsicles. Full. And these little bags weren't uniform shapes because the milk wasn't solid when I put them in there. They froze into warped little statues sagging between the grills of the freezer shelves or smushed up against a pack of peas or around a can of orange juice concentrate. It was way too late by the time

I figured out I should have stacked them flat to save space. I was also beginning to run out of bags and those little plastic clips that sealed the tops.

Sean and I decided it was time to try and have Erin drink from a bottle now that we seemed to have the nursing thing down. It would free me up a little (although I was still uncomfortably full of milk most of the time, so I still had to pump every few hours) and maybe cut into the supply in the freezer a little. She would have none of it. No matter how carefully we warmed the milk, she knew that silicone nipple wasn't mine. I swear, even if I left the room when he tried to coax her to drink a little, the second I returned she began screaming at me and my hormones took over. Just the sound and sight of her hungry little self triggered a milk letdown that soaked my Heavy Absorbency Kotex to dripping. One night I went out for a few hours hoping that she would eventually get hungry enough to give in, but when I came home way past her feeding time she had outlasted Sean and we both felt so guilty we gave up. And the bags of frozen breastmilk multiplied into the hundreds.

One weekend, my in-laws came for a visit and we began to realize that our world had changed significantly. Most of the time I kept the heavy breast pump in the living room so that I could use it several times a day while reading or watching television as I nursed. In preparation for the visit, we moved it to our bedroom which meant that I disappeared every few hours for a while to pump and nurse. I often fell asleep while nursing and was gone for a lot longer than I had planned to be. It was during one of these times that my very conservative father-in-law headed into the kitchen to get a glass of ice water. He opened the freezer door and was instantly pelted by a dozen or more sliding breastsicles cascading out of their precarious perches. Sean ran over to explain what these strange little packets were and the freezer stayed firmly shut for the remainder of their stay.

It wasn't long before the milk started to go bad. If you haven't ever smelled rotten human breast milk, I don't encourage it. It is the most foul, most spoiled-smelling substance and can turn even the most iron of stomachs. It smelled so bad that I, a tree-hugging, granola-eating, recycling fanatic from Oregon, stopped even removing the little plastic clips from the bags before throwing them away. I, who could have found a million other uses for those handy little plastic pieces and lamented their ten-thousand year stay in a landfill near me, who had cleaned up vast oceans of vomit and debrided septic wounds without gagging, couldn't bear the smell of my own sour breast milk. I tossed those nasty little bags without even opening them up. Each and every one.

Eventually I was able to give up the breast pump by gradually decreasing the amount I pumped off and then the number of times I pumped during the day. I suffered multiple bouts of mastitis and severely clogged ducts over the course of a few months, but I was suffering from some serious cabin-fever and I was tired of being tied to that damn machine all day long. Spending nights with a hot washcloth pressed to my sore, stopped-up breasts was worth it if I could just leave the house for more than an hour at a time.

And finally it happened. Erin and I figured out how to breast-feed without any special accessories or techniques and I decided it was time to take a girlfriend up on her offer of a lunch date.

Kendra loved babies and was considering getting pregnant, so our first few minutes consisted of her cooing over Erin. We finally settled in across the table from each other near a window and a young twenty-something college boy came to take our drink order. As soon as he left, Erin started fussing and I decided to show off my mad nursing skills. I turned toward the window, my back to the dining room, whipped out a towel to cover my shoulder and breast and tucked Erin discreetly beneath it, unhooking the clasp on my bra and letting her root in to find my nipple. She quickly latched on and I said a silent prayer of thanks to the Nursing Goddess above. My milk started gushing almost instantly and the baby greedily gulped it down.

Unfortunately, Erin had recently hit that milestone where she was visually interested in everything around her and she began waving her little arm to dislodge the towel tent she was trapped beneath. With one arm supporting the baby, I had to repeatedly tug the top of the towel back over her head as she kept swatting at it. Even though it was February, we were both sweating with effort in minutes.

The cute young waiter chose that moment to return with our drinks and I turned my body slightly more toward the window to conceal the rapidly sliding towel. I craned my neck back to look at him so he would know we were ready to order just as he clapped his hands together with a peppy, "What can I get for you ladies today?"

The clap startled Erin just as the towel slid off of her sweaty head and she swiveled her head to look up at him. Her mouth followed the trajectory of her eyes, pulling away from my breast which, in addition to being now fully exposed, was in complete "letdown mode." Because my body was still under the impression that it was entirely normal to release breast milk at 150 pounds per square inch, an Old Faithful-worthy geyser of milk shot out onto the window next to me, hitting so hard it splashed back onto the table and cascaded in a waterfall down onto the windowsill. I barked, "ERIN!" and tried desperately to guide her mouth back to the shower of milk but she would have none of it. It felt like hours before I was able to retrieve the towel and cover myself. By the time I looked up, Kendra was shaking with silent laughter, tears in her eyes, and all that remained of the waiter was the dust cloud he left behind as he retreated.

We didn't see him again. A few minutes later, with Erin settled quietly back in her car seat, a lovely woman came to take our lunch order as if nothing had ever happened. I cleaned the sticky mess off of the window the best I could with the already-saturated burp towel and hoped that someone would come by soon to do a more thorough job before it soured and stunk the place up.

BREASTFEEDING BOOT CAMP

ANNA BRAFF

W HEN I WAS PREGNANT I always assumed I would breastfeed, never contemplating that it would be challenging or downright difficult sometimes. Breastfeeding seemed like the natural, obvious and logical choice one makes as a mother to start her child off right. My long-term objective is to breastfeed my son, Evan, for at least one year, but as a first-time mother, I've found that no one really prepares you for breastfeeding boot camp. No preparatory program exists for adequately learning the ropes. The basic introductory courses you take—perhaps with your partner, too—cannot really prepare you for the bumps in the road. If you are lucky, you get a baby who is not fussy on the breast or does not have vacuum-like sucking capabilities.

Early on, my son had a vice grip on my boobs when he wanted to feed. It was painful! We suffered from latching issues; we were not mastering the "deep latch" technique instantaneously like I was *told* I should. It was beyond an unpleasant experience and it resulted in chapped, cracked, dry, and yes, bloody nipples. I thought, "How could something so natural be so painful?" I refused to give up, so I hired a lactation consultant. Hiring a lactation consultant is synonymous with modesty being passé. Childbirth certainly primed me for being shamelessly naked in front of strangers, but breastfeeding cemented it.

Samantha was my lactation consultant. She was a very sweet and knowledgeable woman, and she only wanted to empower me to continue my breastfeeding journey. In order for her to help me I was required to sign release forms allowing her to touch my breasts. Prior to her arrival, I was quite naïve about what would actually happen. I signed the consent forms and she asked me to demonstrate how I latched my baby for breastfeeding. I asked, "Do I just remove my breast and show you?" Of course! How else would someone help you with breastfeeding? Feeling slightly sheepish, I threw caution to the wind and whipped out a boob. Of course, my work-from-home husband witnessed everything, as did my mother-in-law, who was staying with us to help us care for the baby. Not that they hadn't attended an exclusive showing in the delivery room, but I thought that part was over. Demonstrating my improper breastfeeding techniques center-stage before a stranger, my new baby, husband, and mother-in-law definitely felt awkward and uncomfortable.

Samantha placed her hand in a surgical glove and began to help me with latching, often touching my breasts. At this moment I realized my boobs were not designated for my husband or me; they were for baby. Having breasts reminds you that you are a sexy woman. I sighed as that sexy feeling associated with having a sensual body hastened. I was in boot camp for a reason. I was training for the most important task: nourishing my baby. Once again, and with trepidation, I guided my son to my breast to latch and it was actually toe-curling. Samantha wanted to see which props I used to aid in nursing. I owned two breastfeeding pillows, which I had purchased on separate occasions. She thought My Brest Friend was the best choice for optimal results. She then stacked several other silk pillows from our couch underneath for added support. We tackled football hold, cradle and cross-cradle. Even the baby grew sleepy after nearly two hours in the thick of breastfeeding boot camp. Eventually my consultant departed to visit other stressed out, lactationally challenged mothers, and I was left alone to confront the challenge with my new bag of tricks.

It certainly *seemed* like my techniques progressed during

the session, but when Samantha left I felt like Dumbo unable to fly without his magical feather. Nevertheless, I persevered. That weekend felt like running on the steepest incline of an endless treadmill. Several people dispensed well-intentioned advice such as, "Just give him formula," or, "Breastfeeding is not the most important thing." I felt like a ping-pong ball, unable to decide what to do. Something told me not to quit and to keep going, so I kept on trying—over and over—and fighting through the pain. My at-home training consisted of one successive latching after another. My focus was to overcome this challenge in the name of health benefits for my son. As the weekend drew to a close, I still did not feel confident. I wavered. "Do I just throw in the towel and give the baby formula?" As the cast of Seinfeld might say, "Not that there is anything wrong with that!"

On Monday, I called Samantha and debriefed her on my weekend. I requested a follow-up session. These consultations were not cheap, but if it meant mastering this skill I rationalized it was well worth it. We made an appointment for the following day. When Samantha returned, I assembled my breastfeeding pillow fortress and latched Evan on to my breast, still feeling that cringing pain. However, as he nursed it hurt less and less. I demonstrated my savvy breastfeeding techniques before Samantha's eyes. She told me that my whole demeanor had changed and that I was a new woman from what she saw at the close of last week. That gave me hope and a spring in my step. Maybe it was worth moving forward with breastfeeding and not giving up? It still hurt, but at least I knew things were improving. It wasn't just me.

The only missing ingredient in the whole breastfeeding experience was someone telling me in so many words, "This is breastfeeding boot camp. It's going to hurt, but it will get better. Nothing is wrong with *you*." It took a good four weeks before Evan and I were copacetic. Following the purchase of several healing ointments, numerous pumping sessions, breastfeeding pillows, covers, accoutrements and lots of practice and tears we finally achieved breastfeeding nirvana.

Since that point, I now breastfeed in any position and no longer use a cover; the shroud of shame is packed away. With my newfound confidence, I breastfeed before mixed company in baby classes and when hanging out with our friends; in public parks and mall parking lots while in my car; in front of our male pediatrician and my in-laws. I've breastfed in so many different places that it is difficult to keep track of them all. Modesty and shame are relics of the past. These ups and downs have shaped me into the proud breastfeeding boot camp graduate that I am today. I wouldn't have it any other way.

BARE WITH ME

SARAH CAMPBELL

WHEN YOU BEGIN TO BREASTFEED, the key is the latch. It's all about the latch. At first, it's not the quality of the latch, but whether or not the newborn is able to achieve that contact. Once the baby has fastened on, and the cloister of breathless midwives and mothers gathered can catch their breath, the real work for you sets in. After the combined time of nursing my two children, I have thought that if only my breasts could have worked in the same way as a coffee maker, halting percolation when the carafe is not there, life would have been simpler, and never would there have been a day when I found myself stuffing my nursing bra with newborn diapers or tea towels.

Please, bare with me.

It is the first week your partner has returned to work, leaving you wearing one of his old t-shirts and a pair of track pants at the front door. Both of your mothers have returned home and the midwives won't be visiting again. You close the door and let out a sigh of relief, looking forward to the restoration of some sort of normal. You turn around and spot your tiny new bundle, lovely and asleep in her bouncy chair in the front room of your home. You think, we can do this, we're going to be just fine. You pick up your child and bring her to the couch where together you sit and cuddle. Around you are a few empty mugs, flannel receiving blankets, a half-empty glass of orange juice, a bran muffin with one bite out of it, a tube of nipple cream, and a bottle of Tylenol. You look into your baby's face, now awake with rosy cheeks, and you watch in awe at the tiny petal lips making sucking movements back and forth. You know it's time. You look around at the heavy curtains still closed against the morning light, use your free arm to lift the t-shirt up and off, pull down the flap of your nursing bra, and bring Baby to breast. You tug at the blanket on the back of the couch and try to get it to cover your bare shoulders. Good enough. Your baby is cradled in the nook of your left arm and using your right hand, you hold your hard, full breast up while pulling your baby in, just like the midwife suggested. You watch the miracle of recognition as Baby's mouth opens and begins to feed. You jump at the contact, a slight pull and pinch, which startles Baby and sets her to tears. You jump to your feet and start to do the walk-and-bounce-dance that all mothers everywhere not only know, but continue to do in grocery store lines for years after their children have graduated from high school.

Baby settles and you return to the couch, wrapping the blanket once again around you. This time contact is made without fail and Baby is happy to nurse and rest her eyes while you lean your head back and do the same. You feel the strong pull of much-needed sleep but sit up, wondering if a little TV wouldn't help. You look around the room and spot the remote at the other end of the couch, a three-seater. *Why couldn't we have settled on the loveseat*, you wonder as you lean to your right, trying not to disturb Baby. Leaning isn't going to do it, so you scooch your bum over just enough to reach the remote when you bump one time too many and the latch breaks. Baby looks around, dazed and lets out a wail. You sit there, for what seems too long, wondering if you should grab the remote. But then guilt kicks in and you shift back to the far side of the couch where you begin to soothe Baby with gentle shushes until she goes back to her meal. You watch Baby feeding away, so peaceful, snoozing against your warmth and again you feel the calm, spreading tide of sleep you have been longing for. You're not sure if sleeping right now is the best idea, you feel you should be awake and folding laundry or baking something at the same time, if you could only figure that out. Your body is begging, tugging at you to let go and sleep along with your babe. You give one last furtive look around the room for a magazine or book to keep you awake and then you give in. You sit forward just enough, gentle enough, and then allow yourself to sink back into the cushions. Your head rests just so and the last thing you think, before drifting away, is how perfect these moments really are. You feel your breathing together with Baby's, just as it had been for those nine months. Your arms encircle her and you're off, asleep. Until thirty seconds later when the doorbell rings and someone is banging on your front door. Baby startles, little monkey arms spasming akimbo. The latch between you is broken and she screams as your milk continues to spray into her eyes. You jump from the couch and throw your right hand over your nipple to contain the milk. You look around the room for something to cover yourself with, all memories of the receiving blankets and burping cloth on the coffee table lost from your mind, and you grab a diaper. You open the stiff diaper and stuff it against your aching breast, which is now lined like a road map with pulsing blue veins, and your child screams as the doorbell continues to ring. You forget that you are without nerdy t-shirt, and march to the front door as a mama bear might approach the entrance of her cave after having hibernation interrupted. You swing open the wooden door, Baby perhaps now shocked into interested silence and you glare at the man who stands before you, wide-eyed, holding out a brown box in his hand. "Amazon delivery?" he asks, frightened. And in the way only a brand new, nursing, sleepless mother can do, you look down and see your babe fast asleep in your arms and in less than thirty seconds you forget it all and your mood switches from crazed to elated.

CARYN LESCHEN

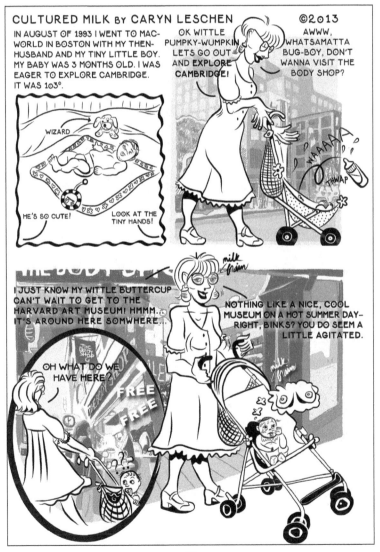

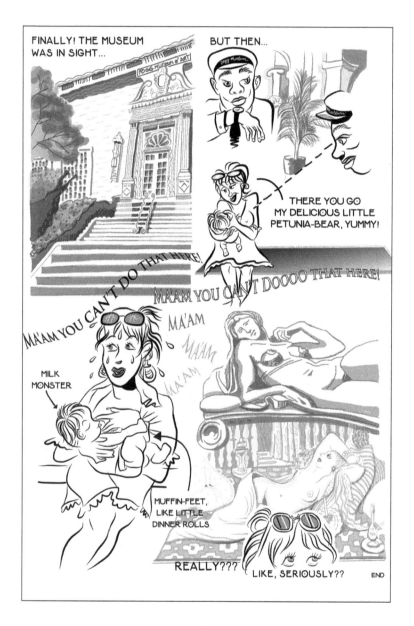

BREAST DRESSED

JENNIFER ANDRAU SHPILSKY

IT STARTED WITH A DRESS, no, a wedding with a need for a dress. It was to be my first official event out since the birth of our second son Willem, but I had one problem...
I had been dutiful, bordering obsessive, when it came to researching the bottomless pit of baby-related knowledge the first time around, so that by the time our second child was on the way, I felt confident I could keep the books on the shelves. Of course I panicked in those last weeks leading up to his arrival and in a frenzy started combing through the basics again. In those last few days of voraciously trying to acquire and file away the little tidbits of information that I would be able to draw on in middle-of-the-night subconscious moments of crisis I never came across that really important bit on bottle-feeding. The one that says that even if your child takes the bottle in the beginning, it doesn't mean he always will. In the midst of engorgement issues and blocked ducts I didn't have time to consider that a spontaneously disappearing bottle wouldn't necessarily be readily accepted again some days or even weeks later. No, it was *not* like riding a bike. My sweet colic-free angel baby had a flaw! In fairness, it wasn't his flaw but his perfect design. He wanted his nourishment the way nature had intended. It was my flaw, my mistake! Being so wrapped up in the world of breastfeeding I forgot to read the tips on bottle-feeding and, like my mother-in-law said, that bottle was my ticket to freedom, freedom to attend a good friend's wedding *sans* baby for a night.

I was about six weeks post-partum when my sweet husband took me shopping for some new clothes and my eyes fell on the most perfectly beautiful dress, a long floral, delicate and feminine. I decided there and then I *would* be going to this wedding and I *would* be wearing that dress! I knew from my grit and determination to get our first child to nurse naturally (six weeks of tears, frustrations, and nighttime fumblings for silicone shields) that a strong resolve and some patience goes a long way. Willem's bottle woes would be solved, that was assured. What I didn't know was exactly *when* this was going to happen and, well, this momma had a timeline. No, it wasn't a timeline to return to work. It was simpler. It was a timeline to have one night away with my husband. A night to be reminded of my femininity and individuality outside of my children.

I can say now that this dress I hawkishly spotted in the department store took on a life as more than a merely beautiful swath of fabric. It really represented the way I wanted to feel inside, that after weeks of exhaustion and leaked milk and endless after-birth stuff, to put it discreetly, I was ready to feel put together and attractive again. The feeling started to bubble up when I tried it on. Insert breast pads, pretend they aren't there, zip, now hesitantly turn towards the mirror. I was prepared to accept the reality of it losing its appeal on my post-partum body, but miraculously, it held its beauty. I just stared. It surely was a magical dress!

I brought it home and just admired it on the hanger for a few days before I mustered the courage to try it on once again. Is it possible I lost weight that quickly? I must have. So, off I went to the store again for a smaller size. It took two women to help me squeeze into that smaller size. After a few perspiration-inducing moments (you know that moment when the zipper has reached a seam and you hold your breath, fearing that a little too aggressive zippering will eat into your flesh), they finally got the zipper up and convinced me that the only

way that dress would stay up over my milk-laden b
to go with this smaller size. It was a questionable r.
they said that I'd probably lose more weight. Musi
ears and so I greedily gobbled up the logic.

Back at home the dress sat again for a few weeks. During that
time we were making a snail's pace in progress with the baby
and his bottle strike. The little man didn't fuss much. On the
contrary, it was a peaceful strike. He played with the nipple,
teasing us at first into thinking he'd take it, but ultimately
spitting it out in defiance of our absurd notion he should drink
from anything other than me. Before I knew it the event was
upon me and the weight loss had clearly slowed. I still needed
a virtual entourage of women to get me zipped up in the dress
and for the first time I realized that, even though I would be
able to enlist my husband to help me into the dress at home,
I would be solely responsible for getting myself in and out of
it at the wedding. Now I don't typically de-robe at weddings
but I was going to have to pump. That was a fact.

There are two things I really despise in life: one is pumping
gas and the other, you guessed it, is pumping milk. I could
come up with a list of other things I despise that would most
definitely be at the top of a "despised-things list," like people
who spit in public or being in earshot of my husband eating
chips, but it's totally off topic and, well I just really need to
dramatize how much I hate pumping for the sake of your
compassion. But, for how much I despise suctioning plastic
cones to my breasts and the ensuing vision of myself on the
dairy farm that comes along with it, there is nothing that will
get me running faster to do so than the feeling of painfully
full breasts, for that is what I would have if I couldn't get that
dress on and off on my own.

Back at the store I tried to resolve the almost impossible situation of needing a dress when I was between sizes. And this
is where I want to interject and sing, no shout, the glorious
praises of the British sizing system because when I walked

over to the dress section and discovered that a size 3 existed in between that 2 and 4, I knew I was going to wear my lovely, beautiful dress after all.

As if on cue little Willem decided he, too, was ready for some resolutions. It could have been due to the suggestion I not come home for a feeding or to us finally choosing the right combo of bottle and nipple from the ever-growing bottle, nipple and pacifier store that had spontaneously sprung up in my kitchen. Whatever the case, there was a brief moment of guilt quickly brushed aside to be replaced with that grit and determination I remembered really only in theory. Sigh. Well, worst case, I'll be home a little after the attempted bottle-feeding to beg his forgiveness with a swiftly-placed breast in the face. Miraculously, though, the pieces all fell together and good thing for that because it really had come down to the wire. But I'm an optimist and had never considered it wouldn't happen, or at least for sanity's sake never allowed myself to consider it. So, it seemed, we would be going to the wedding after all.

The day arrived and even though most of the major details had been ironed out I had a sense of dread. Some things I had to resign to chance but those things fed my anxiety. When should I pump exactly? Would I do it coinciding with the baby's feeding? The way I calculated the timing it seemed to not be an option, as the bride and groom would most likely be in the middle of vow exchanges. More importantly, where would I do it? At the wedding? It was an outside garden wedding. At the reception? I had never been to the place and had no idea of what to expect. In a dark corner? In the car? In the car in a dark corner? In a bathroom? What do you do? Sit on the toilet? I saddled up my husband with the pump and donning my beautiful masterpiece of a dress headed out the door. The freedom was overwhelming. Instantly I felt like I had forgotten something. Did I leave my phone? No, I had that. Was it my lipstick? No, it's right here. Oh right, the kids, particularly that three-month-old who just taught himself that silicone was his best friend in mommy's absence. What if he changed his mind? Well, to hell with all the questions. We'd swing it. I say "we" because I told myself my husband was in on this, too, for solidarity's sake, but let's face it, ladies, when it comes to stuff like this we are pretty much on our own. We are left to our own devices, to chance and, optimistically, to unexpected acts of generosity from complete strangers.

The wedding ceremony was beautiful and as I held back tears watching the beaming groom watching his stunning bride make her way down the aisle, I felt that first letdown. I looked down and noticed my breasts had decided to double in size at which point they were no longer a fan of the dress that held them back. I was bordering on obscenely inappropriate cleavage. Neon flashing lights might as well have been hung over me. Check out the hussy in the second to last row! Don't let that sweet floral print fool you! Thank goodness this was a wedding ceremony and all eyes were on the lovely couple but I still couldn't help the paranoia. I needed to get strapped to my dairy pump and fast. At last the couple made their way down the aisle and it was time to head to the reception. With feigned timidity I politely motioned for a couple nearby to exit into the aisle before me, when all I really wanted to do was push them aside and tear down the aisle with my dress gathered up in my arms. Mustering the decorum that was required of me upon seeing familiar faces on the way out I managed to artfully hide my pained expression in the occasional obligatory salutation of airy cheek kisses.

In the short drive from Beverly Hills to West Hollywood though, there was enough time to feel yet another flood of milk course down my chest. In that time I got the text I was anxiously awaiting. Our sweet angel man was fast asleep at home, unaware of my body's store of milk being prepared for him. Willem clearly had no qualms with silicone tonight.

Pulling up to the reception, I quickly realized that pumping in the car was not an option. All cars were being valeted and, well, there were people for miles. I breathed an equal sigh of relief and dread. Thank goodness the car was not an option for I really did not see how one could be discreet while wearing a zippered strapless gown, but what now? Enter above-mentioned generous stranger. She swooped in like an angel of mercy. She had to have been. Really, what twenty-something West Hollywood actress/waitress compassionately delivers a severely lactating mom, naively parading around in a designer dress, from her body's natural yet painful response to untapped milk? And the speed with which she whisked me away! It was unprecedented kindness. I mean, I had hardly heard the request escape my husband's lips. Really? Who were these people? My husband? This woman? Is it possible that I wasn't alone in all of this? I was led silently to a back office past the bathrooms, past the kitchen, winding our way through the maze of hallways in what felt like a covert operation. We moved swiftly with just a rustle of fabric our only evidence of existence. It's possible though if some quick-reflexed kitchen staff had looked up in time he might have caught a piece of floral fabric in his left field of vision. At last we arrived. I had the small room all to myself. I was told the door locked automatically and only two people had the key, the angelic actress and the manager. Wait, you said *he*, right? Okay, yes, please *do* tell him I'm in here. Wine? Why yes! I'll have some wine. Water, too? Are you sure it's no trouble? There I sat with my glass of wine, glass of water, the pump before me, and the moment upon me. I had made it. No, not on my own. With the help of others. But wait, it wasn't over. I needed to actually get out of this dress, pump without spilling, zip myself back into the dress and get back to the party. Alright, here I go.

I reached down to set up the pump and stopped. I hesitated not knowing what to do first, set up the pump or undo the dress? Deep breath! You made it. Relax. Have a sip of wine and just enjoy the fact you have it this good, that you aren't pumping in a back alley nervously looking over your shoulders for any potential voyeurs who also happen to have a really obscure fetish of watching women pump milk out of their breasts. Okay, *now* here I go.

Crap! Where's the tubing? Oh my god. All this effort and my husband left the tubing at home! I could just cry, polish off this wine, and then cry some more. After all of this I will have to go home now? Wait! Oh thank goodness. For crying out loud, get a grip woman. He had just zippered it up in the bag. I just have never seen the bag so neat, all the pieces tucked away. Bless that man's type A-ness.

I proceeded to expertly join piece after piece and finally insert the tubing. Carefully setting the contraptions down amongst hand-written notes to order particular wines and stacks of fine dining resumes, I turned my attention to the dress. Undoing the top hook I unzipped hesitantly. I realized my vulnerability. Under bright office lights in a strange room in a very public place, I had to completely undress down to my waist, and in such a bold way. It was not like I could just lift a shirt. The whole top half had to come on down. Folding over the bodice of my dress, I prayed that no one would come bursting through the door. At that moment, I glanced over my shoulder and noticed for the first time the video monitor on the wall. There was the party, everyone milling about enjoying their cocktails. This was kind of nice. There's what's-her-name. I really need to catch up with her. I'll figure out her name first and then go talk to her. Who's that guy again? He looks familiar. Hmm. I'll have a sip of wine, make a little virtual toast. It's like I'm practically there, only I'm half-naked! At first I felt like I was milling about the party in the nude. It took my reptilian brain a few seconds to catch up to technology and slowly convince itself that I was not exposing my lactating breasts to all the party-goers I could see.

Clad in floor-length floral fabric from the waist down and bare from the waist up, I proceeded to suction on the pump shields. For some reason, I had not gotten the memo on the ins and outs of double-pumping and was resigned to self-punishment by holding both pumps, one in each hand, perfectly aligned while willing myself to ignore the occasional itch from hair strands falling onto my face. It's not like I hadn't heard of this miraculous bra that holds everything on for you. It's just that I thought I didn't need it. I didn't need it like I need water, food and sleep, but want can definitely border on need when it comes to products like hands-free pumping bras. I learned that quickly. Even so, I managed some incredible feats that evening. I'm pretty sure my elbow spawned a hand at some point allowing me to pump while taking an occasional sip of wine and even sending out a text to a friend reveling in the fact that I *had* three hands.

I managed to enjoy my awkwardly rigid position with a view to the outside world, and just when I started to relax (as much as I could in that position) I looked up and noticed the security camera in the top corner of the ceiling. Before I could even process what I had seen, my natural defensive instincts ignited a spark in my legs that swung me around in my swivel chair to face the back wall away from the prying eyes of the camera. Paranoia quickly overcame me, and, while I'm sure I had complete privacy in that room, I couldn't rule out that my guardian angel actress/waitress had overlooked the possibility that my room was being broadcast for a slightly amused audience elsewhere—maybe those kitchen guys for one. Sigh. It was over. I was no longer a virtual part of the party. It was nice while it lasted. Anyway, I think I'll give myself another five minutes and return to the real party praying I don't get any knowing looks or worse, averted eyes from the wait staff.

At last I deemed enough milk had been extracted to provide me an enjoyable rest of the evening. I set my pumped milk aside and started to unscrew parts, entrusting my slightly cortisol-infused limbs to not spill any of that amazing liquid gold. Nope, not a drop. Now I just needed to get back into my dress and rejoin the party. The milk tucked away next to an ice pack, I turned my attention to getting dressed. Straighten out breast pads, put on strapless bra and zip up dress. Crazy, flesh-eating zipper moment avoided and, phew, this momma was back in business! Now it was done! I was done! I reached down for the little black backpack, my glass of wine (the water could stay) and headed out the door. There was just one last pit stop, the bathroom, and I would be on my way. I touched up my lipstick and walked out. I felt a huge weight lifted off my shoulders, or breasts rather, as I walked out of the bathroom door gleefully clutching my glass of red wine. And that's when it happened. The door was just a tad heavier than I had calculated, or I might have been too excited to get back to the land of adult conversation, but either way, that heavy wooden door came closing down fast and hit my wine-bearing arm hard. My heart stopped as I watched red wine being propelled forward in slow motion. Oh, for the love of it all! Wine splattered the floor in front of me and in that moment, surprisingly, an unprecedented calm set in. Maybe it had to do with the slightly camouflaged nature of floral pinks and purples or maybe I tapped a higher motherly power, but I calmly headed back into the bathroom, commenced with a little dabbing and walked back out as if nothing had happened. I found my husband and seamlessly joined the conversation. In the flash of a moment, our eyes met to confirm that it had been a success. A slight nod of my head and a knowing look, a secret language shared between spouses, confirmed that I had mentally survived the day's unknown mommy adventure. Still, he had no intricate knowledge of the pumping endeavor I had just enjoyed, the fumbling, the fear of being unknowingly watched, and the splattered wine. That was a story for later. For now it was time to laugh and dance.

I could not have planned it any better, because, well, I didn't. Sometimes chance works out better than anything we could ever plan. Strangers and loved ones surprise us and in the end, a little caution gets thrown to the wind.

FROM HERE TO THERE

JESSICA CLAIRE HANEY

I T WAS GOING TO BE THE PERFECT GETAWAY. For a few hours, anyway. The resort near my in-laws' place in Vermont was purported to be beautiful, a haven even if you're not a nursing-around-the-clock mother of a five-month-old who just cut his first tooth. At the end of our visit, my sister-in-law, mom to a two-month-old, was going to join me for an afternoon of respite from the feed/change/jiggle and nurse-to-sleep routine.

Now all we had to do was get there. Driving up from our home outside Washington, D.C., we stopped for an overnight at my sister's house in New Jersey. In our limited time as parents, we'd spent almost all our driving hours tuning out screams, unless we drove at night. After dark, it was quiet—on the road, and in the car—but tiring.

On our first attempt putting rubber to the road to visit my parents a month earlier, we'd figured out that giving our son a bottle was a lot speedier than stopping, unstrapping, and nursing a slow feeder. But I was a stay-at-home mom without much milk supply, in my breasts or in the freezer. One-sided pumps didn't work for me, so I planned to bring the full Pump 'N Style on vacation so that I could provide our baby's drive-time snacks and his feeding while my sister-in-law and I luxuriated in the spa and finally got some exercise at in the resort's fitness center and yoga studio.

Shortly before we planned to leave New Jersey, I got the pump out of the trunk. I'd carefully planned to pump out the foremilk for the bottle on the road and then, just before we left, nurse my son with the fatty hindmilk so he'd zonk out in the car seat for the first few hours.

I lugged the black bag over my shoulder to the well-used couch in my sister's sunken family room and found an outlet behind a lamp to plug it in. Up I flipped the Velcro top, which held the supplies and my not-even-close-to-sexy bustier. My sister's daughters had been around a lot of nursing moms, but not a lot of pumpers, so I felt like something of a zoo attraction. "Here's how it works, girls! You, too, can aspire to be a mom trying to cobble together a sense of sanity while providing for your children."

I zipped up the white cotton so that only my small, pale nipples and a little flesh showed through, but when I went to wedge in the plastic trumpets, they weren't there. "Where are the flanges?" I cried.

There was no back-up bag of pump supplies where they might be lurking. I'd brought only three bottles total—two for pumping plus one extra—and just the tubes, but nothing to go from the tubes to my boobs and to connect my boobs to the bottles. The long plastic hoses just hung limp, like snakes without a mouth.

My heart sank. How could I be so stupid to leave the pump parts at home? My mind fast-forwarded to my planned day of escapism suddenly slipping out of my reach. My son was both a frequent and a long, lazy nurser. Without a bottle, it seemed impossible to imagine that I'd be able to enjoy more than about 75 minutes of leisure time in the middle of the day before I knew my enjoyment would be at my boy's expense. But I so wanted a massage! And I needed the exercise! If I could just have a few hours, I thought, maybe then I could feel centered, calm, happy. For weeks, I'd been imagining myself emerging from this vacation ready to be the mother I'd dreamed of instead of the stressed-out specimen I'd become. Without the pump, bliss was slipping through my fingers.

My nieces looked at me with disappointment and confusion, like I was a giant "out of order" sign.

"There's a Babies 'R' Us that's not really out of your way," my sister offered. She got out a map, and we pondered the merits of taking a back road to spend a bunch of money on something we didn't really *need*. Despite my firm decision not to work outside the home for at least another year, I convinced myself that someday it might be worth having two sets of trumpets. And I did want to get a gift for my new niece...

So off we went, in the dark of night, in search of a brightly lit oasis of all things baby, the gateway to my lactation vacation. I stayed in the parking lot with the back door slightly ajar, nursing the baby good and full for our bedtime drive. John emerged not long after with a white and yellow box of overpriced plastic and a Whoozit toy for my son's cousin. Crisis averted.

As it turned out, this detour really ought to have been the least of my concerns approaching our first vacation with baby. I hadn't figured on how challenging it would be to ensure that a child naps while his father is trying to get in a round of golf. But no one enjoys being around an over-tired baby, and since ours wouldn't figure out how to put himself to sleep for another four years or so, I was still on duty, even on location.

For three or four days leading up to the planned spa day, I got increasingly bitter about being saddled with sleep duty, hanging out for hours alone in the hotel room, breast at the ready. The one time I tried to get the baby to nap at my in-laws' in their tiny guest room, he woke up every time I pulled him off, no matter how tired he seemed. Nothing was timed right. On our last full day, when we finally got to the resort—full bottle in tow, thanks to our indulgent, redundant purchase—the window between my arrival and my massage appointment was narrow and gave me just a sliver of time to make it to yoga, which would end right when I'd be famished and ready for dinner. As a nursing mom, my appetite rivaled that of King Kong; my son wasn't the only one who needed to eat around the clock. I had just 45 minutes to work out and shower before my massage. Shortly after I got on the treadmill and looked through the window out over the meadow, intending to clear my head and find a meditative rhythm, there appeared my husband out on the deck, eating a sandwich while my son's head bobbed in the sling. I didn't know if he could see me through the window, but I could sure see both of them. So much for escapism.

Eventually I accepted that nothing is simple when a mom is her child's sole source of nourishment, and there is no escape. Except growing up. And even then, our children will always be connected to us, with no need of any special instrument. "Out of order" doesn't have an entry in the dictionary of parenting.

NIPPOS QUACKING

MICALA GINGRICH-GAYLORD

I HAD WHAT SOME MAY CONSIDER a pregnancy not to be repeated. The story started with the battle of even getting pregnant, riddled with pain and sadness in thinking I was not going to be able to complete what I thought was the most fundamental task: I am a woman, I make a baby. This was to be the first among many surprises about being a woman and a mom and a baby-maker. Once I finally got pregnant, I spent a good portion of the pregnancy on bed rest so that I could complete the all-important task. While on bed rest, I also spent a good deal of time relishing season after season of *The Sopranos*, among a long list of TV shows that made me laugh and cry. My pregnancy and my breastfeeding story begin in a small Midwestern town.

I was not exactly right at home in Middle America, and maybe I felt like bit of an outcast. I am large-boned woman, an artist, tattooed, not a dress-wearing type. Being all those things *and* pregnant made my stand-out factor pretty large. When my daughter Basil was born in October at a whopping five pounds, eighteen inches long, we thought we knew just about EVERYTHING. I was going to be a stay-at-home mom, barefoot, with boobs flapping in the wind and homemade bread in the oven. As it turned out, most of those things did not come to pass. Breastfeeding was something I deeply wanted for her and for myself, but from the outset it was hard—extremely hard. Like so many things about motherhood, I thought it went a certain way ... and the mythology said: baby is hungry, you have food, they eat it. Beautiful images in art tell us that breastfeeding works, our friends seemed at ease with it, and even my own mom talked about how joyful and great it was. Full Halt. Because Basil came early, her tiny mouth was not able to handle my very large boob. You see, I have those baby head-sized boobs, the all-enveloping, come-to-momma kind. But Basil's mouth was the size of half my nipple. This among a few other hiccups added to my high level of stress and feeling like I was failing my baby. So we needed help and we found ourselves at the local hospital after a week at home with little to no success of feeding a very hungry and cranky baby. Fortunately, we had a great program available to us—because as it turns out, breastfeeding can be hard for lots of people. WHO KNEW?

I sat waiting with tiny Basil in my arms, along with Zack, my very kind and tattooed rail of a husband, in a 1990s mauve-colored, low-light room with two chairs and a number of informational posters about being a breastfeeding mother. I had already cried and cursed a few times that morning and was not even sure I could let down milk in this ugly room, let alone be seen as a failing mom in public.

In walked our nurse. She wore a very traditional-looking nurse's dress and smiled kindly at us. She was also wearing a religious head covering and sensible New Balance tennis shoes. It would be prudent to tell you that at this point I was now feeling less than enthralled at the idea of pulling out my very large boob in front of this very proper-looking woman whose wholesome smile and clothing made me feel so very un-wholesome.

When she opened her mouth to say hello, what came out was one of the worst and most extreme cases of a speech impediment I'd ever heard, second only to Elmer Fudd. "Hewow, I yo nuus. How ar yo nippos fewling?" I was speechless and tears were fast forming around my eyes, as she smiled and asked, "Aar you having any quacking, used any wotion on the nippos?" Zack at this point was crying and trying to hold back a torrent of laughter. The nurse in all her sweet Midwestern style was gentle and kind but dear God there was no stopping the laughter that came pouring out of us. She took it in good stride and held my breast to Basil's mouth. What I found in that moment was that humor, a thing that I believe in as the elixir for all things, was allowing me to let down the sweet un-anxious, un-ashamed milk for my tiny baby. With the help of the "nippo guard" Basil began to drink and drink and drink. We were drunk with laughter and she with my milk. As I continued to cry and laugh, my sweet little baby looked up at my bare breast as it sprayed milk all over her. It was a good day to be who I am, and a good day to remember that laughter is in fact the best medicine.

PLUM LACTO

JULEIGH HOWARD-HOBSON

WHEN MY BREASTFED THREE-MONTH-OLD son began to show the unmistakable signs of a yeast infection, I called my wise and knowing midwife to find out what I could do about it. She suggested that, instead of treating the mild infection with antibiotics that could upset his newborn stomach, I should use a time-tested all natural remedy called gentian violet. My husband and I were more than happy to do so, glad to hear that the usual side effects didn't exist with this sort of treatment.

The directions on the little bottle of inky liquid said to liberally swab the gentian violet all over the affected parts. In this case, the parts were my son's mouth. It sounded simple enough. The trick, though, was to fool our three month old into thinking that this medicinal-smelling purple stuff, which we were trying to stick in his mouth with a Q-tip, was no big deal. His initial reaction to our first attempt was to clamp his little jaws closed tight. His second reaction was the same. As was his third.

We decided to go with an alternative method.

We ended up merging feeding (one of his top three activities at the time—the others being sleeping, and using diapers) with treating. I held him up to my breast and he opened his mouth ... then: we swabbed, really really fast, before he could protest with that mouth clamp of his ... I nursed him a little more, then ... I pulled him off, swabbed, then nursed, pulled, swabbed, nursed ... it was fairly easy, once we got the hang of it. We painted the roof of his mouth with one last swab of gentian violet, he had one last nurse and he fell asleep.

Gently ... ever so gently ... I removed him from my breast. I looked down at my slumbering babe. His rosebud lips, his tiny perfect nose, his chipmunk cheeks, his dimpled chin ... were all purple. Vivid, bright, uncompromising, purple.

But, being an eggplant-hued infant notwithstanding, he was sleeping with his mouth closed so that the gentian violet (at least the gentian violet that still remained where we put it) would have a chance to work, before he drooled it all away. My husband and I figured that it was a much better idea to clean him off *after* his nap. Shaking my head at my son's facial purpleness, I looked down at my own chest ... I was bright purple, too. *Glowing purple.*

I put the baby down, and quietly went into the bathroom to wash the purple off. Nothing happened. It didn't come off. Not one bit of it came off. It didn't even tone down. I scrubbed. I rinsed. I re-scrubbed. I used my husband's man-soap! Nothing. No difference. There they were: my two purple breasts topped with two even more purple nipples. I looked like something from a demented version of Dr. Seuss.

Of course, my midwife did tell me to be careful with the gentian violet, before I went out to buy it, because it could really stain. But at the time I just thought she meant it could stain baby bibs ... not people.

I wailed to my husband, waking up my son. My purple-faced son. He looked like an angry plum. When I picked him up and started nursing him, my husband remarked that we looked like a human grape bunch (I stayed married to him anyway).

Nothing, but nothing, would shift the tint. And I tried it all—from oatmeal baths to castile soap. Nope, we were stuck being violet until it finally faded away.

It was a long week. But, at least we can say that we avoided the usual side effects.

THE GIFT THAT KEEPS GIVING

GINA KAYSEN FERNANDES

I NEVER THOUGHT I'D BE ONE of *those* moms. You know the type. The mom with the kid who walks up to her at a park, lifts up her shirt, and asks in a complete sentence if he can nurse. I didn't even know anyone who had nursed a baby past the first birthday. But to my surprise, breastfeeding turned out to be the gift that keeps giving.

Before I became a mom, I thought breastfeeding would be a chore that required herculean effort to nourish my newborn. To my surprise, it was much easier than I imagined, once my sore nipples healed. I quickly saw it for what it really was: a blessing and a simple solution to a wide range of tear-inducing scenarios. Hungry? Check. Tired? Check. Fussy? Check. The boobs have been my go-to utensils that soothed both of us in the most stressful situations.

When my son was four months old, I went back to work. I pumped feverishly in my office to maintain production. I assumed that once I stopped the dreaded pumping after his first birthday, "the twins" would eventually dry up like grapes on the vine. My son would self-wean, just like my friends' babies did, and clutch his sippy-cup with the same enthusiasm he showed when he tugged at my shirt and insisted on his "nana."

But that didn't happen. Pumping or not, the milk kept flowing. As baby grew into toddler, I found that we both still enjoyed it, although the experience and our relationship had changed.

For a toddler, nursing is about the emotional bond rather than basic nutrition. There are times when I felt confined by

95

this emotional crutch. I wanted my breasts back. Couldn't I be a little bit selfish? Hadn't I given enough of my body to pregnancy, childbirth, and now this endless nursing? But then there were the pangs of guilt. If he still wanted the bonding and closeness, why would I take that away? There was also the wistful longing to hold onto my baby just a little bit longer.

But then I got pregnant. It was planned to a tee. We learned the gender, picked a name, and still had all the baby gear in storage. I was completely ready for baby number two but had no clue how to wean baby number one. I read about breastfeeding during pregnancy. It's apparently taboo in most cultures. My mother-in-law grilled me about weaning when I nursed my fussy toddler over Skype. I could harm the fetus, she said. But my OB/GYN was cool with it and assured me nursing would cause no distress.

The growing fetus might have been fine, but I was withering. I was exhausted, nauseated, and impatient with my insistent son who demanded his nana. I tried scaling back the nursing to just naps and bedtime. I refused to nurse in public, mostly because I felt self-conscious. I read blogs about tandem nursing, which kind of freaked me out. Could I really nurse two children at once? The image of a toddler and a newborn baby latched onto my boobs crossed the line for me. I had reached my limit. I had to latch up the bra strap.

And so, after two-and-a-half years, my son learned a phrase: cold turkey. "Mama, I don't like cold turkey!" he cried, when I set the ground rules in no uncertain terms. I laid down the law, and it sucked for both of us. The first refusal was the hardest, but he is a resilient little kid and was soon sleeping soundly without the comfort of my boobs. There were times when he would ask about them. "Mama, I miss the nanas. Can I just take a look?" I would do my best to redirect the conversation and distract him.

To my surprise, I was pretty resilient, too. For more than two years, we'd had this daily relationship and suddenly it was gone for both of us. But I now had the beginning of a new relationship with my growing son. He was less baby to me and more big boy. The older brother was ready for a new arrival.

Once the new baby came, I was back in the saddle. This time, nursing was second nature. Big brother came to accept that his younger sibling would receive the same nana nurturing that he received. Even now, two years since he weaned, he will mention how he misses that closeness. I don't regret the choice I made, but now I must deal with weaning toddler number two. I don't have the excuse of pregnancy. That's not going to happen. So I'll need to get to a place where I feel ready again to reclaim my body for myself without an excuse. Cold turkey may soon reappear on the menu.

DINNER TIME

ADRIANN COCKER

NAKED FROM THE WAIST UP at the dinner table. With my husband. And parents. Giant breasts should be a turn on, but these were far from it. This was my first meal back home in our loft after our son's delivery and I didn't care that my swollen, bleeding breasts were probably not appetizing, to say the least. I needed to eat, and breastfeeding wasn't turning out like I had hoped.

The truth is that I wasn't totally naked on top. I did have on a nursing bra, with clasps undone so that my breasts could air dry (I would have showered with that bra on because of the support and relief it provided!) The hospital nurses recommended the air drying, but I'm betting they didn't have sitting and eating in mind when they gave that handy tip. While I scarfed down my food, knowing that my breasts would be called back into duty at any moment, I contemplated how I even arrived in this situation in the first place.

There was a movie shown in my all-girls high school that showed the miracle of birth. Really it showed some red-faced laboring lady, calmly pushing out a baby in a relatively short amount of time. The infant suckled easily. How hard could this be? I resolved at that time I would have a natural birth and breastfeed my very distant future children.

After that I didn't see anyone nursing in person for almost a decade. When I asked my friend if I could go with her while she nursed her young daughter, I ended up feeling squeamish and turned away. What I should have done is calculated the angles of her arms, asked if the "football hold" worked well for her, and leaned in for a close-up view of the latch when the baby switched sides.

When we were eight months pregnant, we took a breastfeeding class with our local lactation specialists. We saw, among other things, a freshly minted newborn crawl up the chest of her mother to latch, ON HER OWN. And while they made sure to tell us how there might be issues—baby will favor one side, letdown may take some time, the first few days will be rough while your breasts get used to the suction—I was certain in my naiveté that I would be a breastfeeding all-star. I did buy some salve, convinced I'd never open it and would end up handing it down to my next new mom friend.

Naturally the birth plan we had didn't go according to plan. There were drugs. And vacuums. And cuts. I recall asking my very well-respected OB/GYN what the f*** he was still doing down there immediately after my son was born—turns out he was stitching me up. Then a nurse came by to press on my belly—what on earth was she doing? I was so exhausted and in shock that I wasted my skin-to-skin bonding time just bonding, not nursing. The poor thing was so hungry he had trouble latching. And it stayed that way for some time. Good thing I had bought that salve; I used it all.

After the topless dinner, followed by a mostly topless week, I found some lactation experts to come to the house. They helped tremendously. By week two I was eating with a top on and my parents could finally come back over. For meals or just to lend a hand.

MISADVENTURES IN BREASTFEEDING
OR, HOW I LEARNED TO STOP WORRYING
AND LOVE BABY FORMULA

NORINE DWORKIN-MCDANIEL

"SO, ARE YOU BREASTFEEDING?" You get asked that a lot when you're a new mom. It's the kind of question—along with *How much weight did you gain with your pregnancy?* and *Are your nipples chapped?*—that even complete strangers feel is well within their rights to ask if you're toting around a baby. And given everything we know about the health benefits of breastfeeding—the higher IQs, the lower risk for illness, asthma, obesity and diabetes—the expectation was that I'd say *Yes.* Because, of course, I'd be foolish ... make that downright *selfish* ... to deny my baby the precious elixir of breast milk.

Funny, though, how some things are so much more black and white before you actually have the baby. Before I gave birth, I was firmly, completely (some in my family would say insanely and annoyingly) on the breastfeeding bandwagon. Formula? For my baby? As if! Why not just pour the kid a martini and light him a stogy while you're at it?

"You and your sister were formula-fed," my mother would remind me whenever I started going on about my plans to breastfeed till my son was oh, about preschool age. "And both of you girls turned out just fine."

I rolled my eyes. This wasn't the first time we'd had this conversation. I was tempted to remind her that we also slept on our bellies and rode around in cars without car seats or seat belts, and I wasn't planning on doing those things either.

"The World Health Organization recommends a year of

breastfeeding," I said for the umpteenth time through what I hoped looked like a smile, but were actually tightly gritted teeth. "And two years is preferable."

"By all means, try," Mom said. "But if you can't do it, that's fine, too."

If I couldn't do it? That thought never crossed my mind. What was to do? It wasn't calculus (or balancing my checkbook for that matter). Wasn't this what breasts were designed for—I mean apart from attracting the fathers of our children in the first place?

So I was surprised when a friend who was due a few weeks after me mentioned she was stocking up on formula. She'd given up breastfeeding her first child after a month, she told me over steaming decafs. With her second, she wasn't even going to bother. "That stuff's expensive," she griped, digging into her fat-free pound cake.

"Breastfeeding's free," I said, trying to woo her back. "You burn 500 calories a day so the baby weight comes off faster." (The prime mom benefit as far as I was concerned.) Feeling like I was dangling bait, I ticked off a few more bennies I'd heard about: a lower risk for diabetes, breast cancer, and fractures; not to mention the emotional connection with the newest member of your family. "Plus," I said, "it's just so much better for the baby."

"I wasn't into it," she shrugged, and moved on to debating the relative merits of Bugaboos versus Peg Peregos. The subject was closed. But as far as I was concerned, she might as well have been talking about whether it was better to let the baby play with electrical outlets or razor wire. I thought about giving her the freebie can of formula that had shown up in my mailbox. After all, I wasn't going to need it. Sipping my venti decaf, I felt ... yes ... I felt superior. Women who claimed they couldn't breastfeed, I thought smugly, just weren't trying hard enough. Or they were looking for an excuse not to. Meanwhile, I'd taken the breastfeeding class. I'd read the breastfeeding research. I could quote Bill Sears chapter and verse. I knew all the benefits my darling boy would reap. I was prepared—no, make that *determined*—to breastfeed my baby till he said when.

Until ... I couldn't do it. (You probably saw this coming, huh? Breastfeeding till preschool? Ha! We didn't even come close.) Things had started out so well. My newborn latched on within hours of making his debut. There was no hassle, no pain. When the lactation consultant dropped by to check on us, I proudly showed off how we'd gotten the hang of nursing so quickly. I hadn't felt so triumphant since I'd been accepted early decision to Oberlin. Of course, you know the old saying, *Pride goeth before a fall*. Look it up in Bartlett's. You'll find a picture of me, breastfeeding.

In the hospital and when we got home, I nursed constantly. But I quickly realized something wasn't quite right. During baby care and breastfeeding classes, it had been drilled into us that we were to see about six wet and three to four soiled diapers daily. I tracked Fletcher's output with the vigilance of a day trader eyeing the markets. With all that was supposedly going in, there should have been more diapers to deal with. A lot more.

The next morning, in full panic, I beelined it to the pediatrician. "Maybe your milk just hasn't come in yet," was her take on the situation. "But you might have to supplement with formula," she warned. "You know, some women just don't make enough milk."

Not enough milk? No one ever said *anything* about not making enough milk. The breastfeeding instructor, (more like the drill sergeant from *Full Metal Jacket* actually) had um ... *emphasized* the exact opposite.

"EVERY WOMAN. MAKES. ENOUGH. MILK. TO FEED. HER BABY," she'd barked on the first day of class. "GOT THAT?" It wasn't really a question. "PROBLEMS," she continued, "ARE OVERCOME BY WORKING *HARDER!*"

Already firmly on that particular bandwagon, I'd taken her "pep talk" as a goad to the fence-sitters in the class who were still uncommitted. "I KNOW!" I'd wanted to shout out. "I'm with you!" Now I latched onto her words like they were a personal guarantee. Every woman could breastfeed. I was a woman. Ergo, I could breastfeed. It had to happen. Simple logic said so.

Later that day, I was relieved to see that my breasts had ballooned to the size of a Vegas stripper's while I was napping. I took it as a sign that, finally, my milk had come in. Now we could get on track, I thought eagerly, settling into the pillows with Fletcher at my breast. But a day or so later at Fletcher's next well-baby visit, the pediatrician had gone from disinterested to alarmed. "He's lost 12 ounces," she said worriedly. Now I was alarmed. Losing eight ounces or so after birth wasn't unusual. But 12 ounces, she said, was way too much.

I raced back to the hospital's lactation consultant. She watched Fletcher nurse for a bit in her tiny office. She positioned him this way, then that way, first on one breast, then the other. I tell you, my breasts haven't been the focus of so much attention since the summer I hung out (as it were) at the topless beach in Spain.

When the consultant was finally done feeling me up, she diagnosed a weak suck reflex for Fletcher and poor production on my part. A double whammy. "You're going to have to give him formula," she said, popping a nipple on a premixed bottle. You know it's game over when the lactation consultant breaks out the formula. And as Fletcher gulped it down like a ravenous man at an all-you-can-eat buffet, my heart broke for my hungry baby.

Driving home, my diaper bag now filled with formula, I burst into tears. "He ... was ... hungry!" I sobbed to my husband, Stewart. In my zeal to feed my baby the perfect food, I'd practically starved him.

Still, I refused to give up on the idea that I could give Fletcher *some* breast milk. The consultant had sent me home with instructions for taking two herbs—fenugreek and milk thistle—and a high-tech, hospital-grade breast pump. If I took the herbs and pumped every time I fed Fletcher, I might, if I was diligent, she said, increase my milk.

"This is where the hard work comes in," I thought, ready to roll up my sleeves or rather, take off my top. I thought, enviously, of my sister Shari. She'd been like a one-woman dairy farm when her boys were babies. She'd actually stockpiled a several-month supply of breast milk in her freezer with both kids because neither boy could drink it fast enough to keep pace with all she made. After her youngest weaned, she pitched *gallons* of breast milk into the trash.

"If I'd known you were going to have so much trouble, I'd have saved it for you," she said sympathetically.

Now that's a sister. Someone you can borrow a cup of breast milk from when you need it. Still, there's no sense in crying over spoilt breast milk. I'd just have to work harder to make my own. The breastfeeding drill sergeant echoed in my ears: "EVERY WOMAN. MAKES. ENOUGH. MILK. TO FEED. HER BABY." Her words became my personal mantra.

Since I was somewhat unofficially "on leave" from my job as a freelance magazine writer, pumping breast milk became my job. My dining room, where I set up the high-powered breast pump, became my new office. I swallowed my herbs, pumped every time Fletcher downed a bottle of formula and willed my body to cooperate. I didn't care that I looked like a Guernsey cow reading *New York* magazine as two electric pumps pulled and sucked at my boobs. I didn't even care when my very proper father-in-law walked in on me, at the dining room table, naked from the waist up, as the pump whirred along. He promptly spun around, shielding his eyes as if they'd been burned.

"Sorry. Sorry about that. Didn't see you there," he mumbled, making a hasty exit. For a guy with an artificial hip, he moves at light speed when he wants to.

But, really, I was so far past the point of worrying about things like modesty or embarrassment, they were like teeny specks in my rearview mirror. I had a single goal—make milk!—and I went at it with the kind of crazed, single-minded determination that kept the Terminator coming for Sarah Connor long after its cybernetic body had been blown to bits and all that was left was a skeletal arm scratching its way through the ruins.

The drill sergeant said I could feed my baby. She *promised* I could feed my baby. Problems meant I just needed to work harder to feed my baby. Looking back, I don't think I ever worked harder at anything, clothes off or otherwise.

The day I got two full ounces out of my breasts, I did the happy dance around the kitchen, holding up the bottle of milky liquid for all to see. At last! It's working! I can do it! For a brief moment, I felt like a topless Rosie The Riveter.

But the euphoria didn't last. No matter how long I pumped, those two ounces were the most I ever got. And the occasional trickle my efforts were usually rewarded with was just ... depressing. A constant reminder that I'd failed in the most basic responsibility a mother has to her child—feeding him the healthiest food possible.

Even though I felt like I was spinning my wheels, I still vacillated about stopping. The thought lingered: Maybe if I just keep trying! Maybe the next pumping session would fill up the bottle. It's the same kind of obsession that drives gamblers to keep feeding their paychecks into the slot machines a few bucks at a time, convinced the next time they pull the lever, they'll hit the jack pot for sure. But as they say, *insanity is doing the same thing again and again, expecting different results.* Finally, even I had to admit that pumping was like squeezing blood from the proverbial stone. With so much else to do with a newborn, the few drops of breast milk I could squeeze out hardly seemed worth the time. And I confess, I was so bone-tired, I couldn't face getting up at night to pump every time Fletcher ate, especially when it was far easier for Stewart to make up a bottle and feed him while I snoozed. Gradually, lured by the promise of full bottles in the fridge, the security of knowing exactly how much Fletcher was eating and my desperate need for sleep, I succumbed to formula's seductive ease. Don't get me wrong, I felt supremely guilty about stopping. Especially when I'd been so arrogantly gung-ho. I often found myself giving long-winded explanations about why I wasn't breastfeeding—to total strangers in the supermarket checkout line who asked the inevitable breastfeeding question and then were no doubt instantly sorry they did. I assured anyone who'd listen that I had tried my hardest. Honest.

But as I watched Fletcher regain and then surpass his birth weight on formula, guilt and disappointment eventually gave way to relief that at last he was getting enough to eat and thriving.

A couple of years later, I got to interview the chair of the American Academy of Pediatrics' breastfeeding committee for a magazine story. After we wrapped up the interview part, I told her my tale, how desperately I wanted to breastfeed, how frustrated I'd been by the process. I'm not really sure what I was looking for. Absolution? Validation? Assurance that I hadn't completely fucked up my kid's brain and immune system? Maybe all of the above.

"How old were you when you had your son?" she asked me.

"Nearly 40, just six weeks shy of 40."

"You know, women who have their first babies after 38 often don't make enough milk," she told me gently.

Really. Now, *that* would have been helpful information to have when I was beating the Every Woman Can Breastfeed drum and wringing out my breasts several times a day. Okay, so the pediatrician had tried to tell me. But I hadn't believed her. I'd thought it was a cop out. But this ... *this* was medical confirmation that it was age, not effort that made the difference. Not that I enjoyed the reminder I was getting older. But at least now I knew for sure it wasn't for lack of trying. The well was dry. You can't pump what's not there.

I could truly let myself off the hook now. I told her I was thankful for her words. And I was doubly thankful that I hadn't given away that freebie can of formula. After all, that stuff's expensive.

Note: *A shortened version of this story previously appeared in* American Baby *magazine.*

THAT SPRING DAY

ROCHELLE JEWEL SHAPIRO

O N AN EARLY SPRING DAY in 1975, the air heady with honeysuckle, I sat on a bench on The Promenade in Brooklyn Heights, nursing my six-month-old daughter. It was a much bigger deal back then to nurse at all, let alone publicly. But with my loose blouses and my daughter in a sling, I managed to nurse her in subways, supermarket checkout lines, and a Yankees game, and still maintain my dignity.

On the particular day I'm remembering, I'd taken her out of the sling and held her in my arms as she nursed, enjoying her suckling sounds as much as the birdsong in the bushes behind us.

Before long, I saw a tall guy walking, swinging his guitar case, his brown curly hair caught in an updraft from the East River. When he got closer, I recognized him.

"It's Harry Chapin," I said.

At the sound of my voice, my daughter unlatched.

In my glee, I got up to greet him. Even though it was a breezy day, my nipples were so inured from all that nursing, I didn't realize that my breast was exposed. When I reached him, I began to fountain from the untethered breast.

"You're really, really glad to see me, aren't you?" he said, smiling.

Others will remember Harry Chapin as a great folk rock singer, composer, playwright, and activist. But when I think of him, I remember his kindness in the face of my greatest nursing bloop.

THE NURSING SECTION FOR ME, PLEASE!

ROZ WARREN

I TRY TO BE DISCREET. It's not as if I stand up in the middle of a crowded restaurant, rip open my shirt and shout, "EVERYBODY LOOK AT ME!" Instead, I quietly unbutton my top and slip the baby onto my breast. You'd barely know what I was up to. Yet some folks glare at me as if I'm sitting there snorting coke or smoking pot, not feeding my baby. I always want to ask them, "What on earth do you think breasts are for?" But I already know the answer—women have breasts to titillate men. Never mind my hungry baby—the only reason I could possibly be exposing my breasts is to turn on guys!

Nursing my baby is just an excuse—I probably only gave birth to my son so I could display my fabulous milk-filled boobs in restaurants and airports, right? The angry looks tell me that I'm breaking the rules. I'm not supposed to uncover my breasts in public to feed my baby. I'm supposed to uncover them in some guy's bedroom to drive him wild with lust.

Some people feel that nursing is a vulgar and unsightly practice, which ought to be hidden from the eyes of decent people. Look—if you don't like what you see, you've got a neck. Turn your head! No matter how much you glare at me, I'm not skulking off to the bathroom to sit on the toilet or the floor, breathing in stale cigarette smoke and Tidy Bowl fumes as I feed my baby to the pulsating rhythm of flushing toilets.

Would you want to eat in a public restroom? Neither does my son. It's not as if a remotely suitable place is ever provided for nursing in private. Nursing in the bathroom means sitting on the floor with the used tissues and cigarette butts, as other women come in and out and comment on your condition. Blank stares are the norm. The occasional expressions of support and outrage—"What a shame you have to hide away in here to feed your baby!"—are as infrequent as they are appreciated.

Maybe in addition to "Smoking" and "No Smoking" sections, public places can have "Nursing" and "No Nursing" sections. Then the grumps and grouches can be spared the sight of those of us engaged in the most important job there is—taking care of children.

A friend of mine was paid a visit by her grandmother, who came in from out of town to see her great-grandchild for the first time. The baby got hungry. Karen proceeded to nurse him. Grandma was shocked.

"Doesn't it bother you to nurse in public?" she asked (referring, of course, to Karen's own living room).

"Oh no," said Karen. "I love to nurse in public! When there aren't enough people around here, I bundle up the baby and take him out to the airport to nurse!"

That's the right attitude.

BREASTFEEDING RULE 1:
EXPECT (AND EMBRACE) THE UNEXPECTED

ELIZABETH LYONS

I'VE LEARNED OVER THE YEARS that when undertaking the intention to breastfeed, in lieu of asking, "In what public places will I be comfortable breastfeeding?" it would perhaps be more prudent to ask, "In what public place won't I end up *learning* to be comfortable breastfeeding?"

With five kids, including a set of twins and an adopted daughter, I've fed babies in just about every way—and every situation—imaginable. I was determined to breastfeed our firstborn only to be blessed with a child sensitive to absolutely everything I put into my mouth including, I believe, toothpaste. Two years later, I was suddenly a mother to newborn twin boys who, while lovely, ate on opposing every-other hour schedules (and seemingly were of the strong opinion that breastmilk was for the weak, not to mention that it was way too slowly delivered).

Having muddled through these challenges, it was our fourth child, George (the one everyone told me would be easy as pie, simply because he was number four and would have no other choice), who presented me with the greatest of breastfeeding challenges—if for no other reason than that he was the first one I was able to exclusively breastfeed for more than 23 days.

I'll never forget the morning of Sunday, November 7, 2004. I'd been simultaneously anticipating and dreading that day for weeks. November 7 was the day of George's baptism, and I knew that, at some point, I'd have to feed him in church. Given that he was only four weeks old at the time, I'd had nary an opportunity to practice my in-public, sustenance-giving routine, and I didn't think church was the best place to expose everyone to my learning process. I had, therefore, purchased a bottle that really did resemble a breast, planning to pump beforehand and hoping for the best.

I'd practiced with this breast-like bottle contraption before, and it had worked well. So wasn't I surprised when the screw top on this miraculous, albeit slightly inappropriate-looking (especially given our location), invention malfunctioned, spilling its contents all over both George and myself. I don't know which had him screaming more loudly: being held by a stranger who was pouring water on his very bald head or wailing in protest because his mother loved him more than anything but yet not enough to be willing to bare it all right there on the altar!

Many of the memories of breastfeeding (or, at the very least, trying to breastfeed) remain, while others are lost forever in the abyss into which I suppose many of our darkest moments perish. That said, I will never forget this moment in the church, not so much because it was the moment when George was baptized but because it was the moment when, standing on the altar with spilled milk soaking the front of my dress, a screaming newborn, and his three older siblings wrestling for best vantage point, I came to declare the reality that underlies so many of these moments: It Is What It Is.

As it was nearly every Monday through Friday for the following nine months as I picked up my daughter from kindergarten and drove to the empty portion of the school's parking lot where I could scoop up George from his car seat, wedge him in between the steering wheel and myself, and nurse him. Even though I attempted (unsuccessfully) to feed him either just before leaving to pick up Grace or just after returning home, he seemed determined to eat at precisely 12:47 p.m. in the northeast corner of a desolate parking lot underneath the shade of a thirty-foot maple tree. So there we'd sit. Grace recapped

every single moment of her day in unfathomable detail, Jack
and Henry bickered and whined about who-knows-what, and
I took the opportunity to lean my head back while nodding at
Grace's story every 47 seconds or so.

THE BADGE OF NURSING MOTHER

VANESSA DRUCKMAN

TO SAY THAT NURSING didn't come naturally to me would be an understatement. It took me three children to get it right.

I could blame my difficulties with breastfeeding on a post-partum encounter with a Nazi-like La Leche coach. I had waited for her for three hours, gently rubbing the bare chicken legs of my beautiful five-and-a-half pound baby girl whose beautiful brown eyes looked into mine trustingly as I pushed her button mouth against my splayed nipples again and again without success. She just did not seem to have the strength to latch on.

When the lactation consultant finally arrived, she was unsmiling and unapologetic. She watched our awkward coupling for a few seconds and, without asking permission, brusquely adjusted my hold and mashed my daughter's face to my breast. Soon she was grasping my breast and Bella's tiny head, forcefully pushing them together while making "tsk, tsk, tsk" noises in her mouth. I was shaking with exhaustion and emotion, and all my new mother instincts were telling me just to stick a bottle in the mouth of my feather-weight daughter. To diffuse the tension, I stroked at the long hairs on my baby's tiny arms, marveling that I had created this creature.

I turned to the breastfeeding consultant and offered up the perfection of my first child, "Isn't she beautiful? Look at her long soft hairs!" She screwed up her mouth with distaste and said, "It looks more like monkey fur than anything. Except even a monkey could latch on with more skill. You have a lot to learn, little one." I sent her away right then and there, appalled to have received my child's first negative evaluation so quickly. But the truth is that the undiplomatic witch was just an excuse to give free rein to my fear of breastfeeding.

In my first few days of motherhood, I was terrified. Terrified of falling into post-partum depression. Terrified of developing cracked and bleeding nipples like the experienced mothers I knew. Terrified of confronting my naked body, day after day, inhaling all the primal post-labor scents my body was emitting under its nubby hospital gown. Terrified of starving my near-term infant to death, because, after all, how could I possibly create something nourishing enough to keep my child alive? The possibility that I might be able to keep from dropping my baby on her head already seemed like too much to hope for.

I reached for the bottle almost to spite her, but really, it was to comfort myself. The label was right there, guaranteeing the nutritional content my child needed. I shoved my breasts back into my bra and began focusing on the mechanics of bottle feeding. I spent the next year regretting my decision, crippled with guilt that I had permanently eliminated any chance of admission to Harvard by withholding that magical IQ-enhancing, immunity-boosting elixir from her tiny mouth. I wished that I had tried harder, been more thick-skinned. When she strained to breathe during a vicious bout of RSV a few months later, the swollen nipples of the lactating mothers in our infant playgroup all seemed to be pointing at me, the weak and unworthy mother in the room.

Yet, even after all those guilt-ridden months, when I gave birth a second time, to a son this time, I chose not to breastfeed him. "Give him some formula," I told the hospital nurses, "and you can keep him for the night." I wanted to rest up, to get as ready as possible to split myself in two, to pay attention to the potty training of my jealous two-year-old while feeding a newborn. A few weeks later, when he turned colicky and started screaming from 10:00 to 2:00 every night, I regretted my decision, but my locked up breasts had dried up in their under-wire prison. I spent three long months trying to soothe his desperate cries, wishing I still had milk that might have eased his discomfort.

It wasn't until I relinquished all control and had a third child that I finally experienced the peace and joy of breast-feeding. When I walked in from the hospital with the baby, our homecoming couldn't have been more chaotic. Instead of being lovingly deposited in her carefully arranged bassinet, my daughter was unceremoniously deposited, still in her infant car seat, in a corner of the room while the older two children jumped and danced all around me, filling me in with all the events of the past three days. But the chaos put everything in place, giving me the confidence I needed to do what was right for each child.

Breastfeeding became my only escape, my time to bond with my third child. I nestled deep into our family room couch with my perfect little girl baby and other distractions faded to the background as I felt the ancient sweet pull of her tiny mouth. More often than not, our peace was interrupted by my other children, demanding that I pick a winner in some desperate toy dispute. Blissfully trapped amidst the couch cushions, all I could do was shrug and smile, pointing at the nursing baby until they wandered off to play a different game. We all adapted to our new dynamics as a family of five during those first few months, the baby fitting into our family as naturally as she fed from my breast.

Now that my youngest is four, it is those quiet moments spent nursing her in the autumn afternoon glow that I miss the most. My children are a dizzying whirl of activity, only willing to slow down and settle close to me for a few short moments at night when we snuggle up to read before bed. I look at her mouth, filled with baby teeth that will soon be wiggling, and wish I could still cup her tiny little head in my hand as she draws milk rhythmically from my breast. I'm sure those baby days were more hectic than the idyllic moments I nostalgically long for, but those moments of breastfeeding bonding that it took me so long to achieve are my most treasured memories of early motherhood. My hard-earned badge of nursing mother reaped the greatest reward.

A SLOW-N-STEADY BREAST MILK STORY

ANNA G. SILVER

I'M A NATURAL KIND OF WOMAN, the "crunchy-granola" type, as it was called when I was in college. And what could be more natural than breastfeeding? It was never a question for me; of course, I would do it. What I didn't know is that breastfeeding isn't always easy.

My pregnancy, though, had been super easy. As an older first-time mom, I took pride in defying the medical odds: no gestational diabetes, no hypertension, and no bed rest for me. I barely even slowed down at work. The only minor annoyance of my growing belly was my ankles, which in month five, as if in sympathy with my abdomen, ballooned to three times their normal circumference.

So when my water broke two-and-a-half weeks early, I was in high spirits. At 1:30 a.m., I called my doula, while my husband stuffed my "all-natural" birth plan into the suitcase for the hospital.

My spirits began to sink when, ten hours later, I still hadn't gone into labor and, one by one, all my visions for the "natural" birth of my child fell by the wayside. My consolation was that—pumped up with Oxytocin—one epidural, one episiotomy, and another twenty-five hours later, I got to hold my beautiful son in my arms. But I didn't have any milk.

Why no milk? Was it the early arrival? Was it those bloated ankles? Was it my vegetarian diet? Was it my age? The pregnancy had been so smooth that it had erased—no, suppressed—my memory of how difficult it had been for me to conceive in the first place. I had beaten the odds, I told myself. Now, the lack of milk, coupled with exhaustion and the hormonal highs and lows of childbirth, stirred up all those emotions again. Maybe my body was not up to the task after all.

I was given a breast pump in the recovery room and I asked to see the lactation consultant, but not much liquid was coming out from the intended orifices. Maybe my weepy eyes were making up for the difference.

I rented a hospital-grade pump, even as the lactation specialist set me up with the bottle and tubes of a Supplementary Nursing System (SNS). I assumed that the SNS would be temporary, until my milk came in. But my milk didn't come. Back home, between snuggling with my baby and bouts of crying, I researched buying breast milk on the Internet. I had read the literature, so I knew how important breastfeeding was for my child. But a part of me also wanted to prove to myself that I could do it. A week later, when after fifteen minutes of pumping every few hours I was getting only drops, I headed to The Pump Station™ for a consultation. The lactation nurse offered me sympathy, facial tissues, and tips on how to position the SNS tubes. Not willing to risk taking chemical drugs for lactation, I resigned myself to a regimen of the SNS, combined with steady pumping, herbal supplements, and eating lots of cucumbers and millet porridge (folk remedies suggested by friends to reduce my swollen ankles).

The SNS was originally designed for adoptive mothers who want to bond with their infants through nursing. It is made up of a flat-sided bottle with a cleat-like top, which is hung around the neck. Two fine tubes thread through the bottle top. One of those is taped to the nipple on one breast, and the other taped to the other side of the chest. Then the tubes are repositioned for feeding on the second breast. As the infant suckles on the breast, he draws formula through the tube from the bottle. The fineness of the tube and the teeth of the bottle-top cleats control the flow of the formula and help to simulate breastfeeding. But, of course, the suckling of the baby works better than any pump to induce lactation. Just as I had almost given up hope, I began to produce milk. I still didn't have enough, however, to abandon the SNS.

If I had been able to breastfeed naturally, I think I would have had few qualms about nursing in public. I discovered, though, that it is very hard to be discreet with the SNS. Sure, once you've mixed the formula, poured it into the bottle, adjusted the bottle height around your neck, and taped yourself up at just the right angle (if the angle of the tube isn't just so, the flow won't work, resulting in frustration for both baby and mom), you can put the baby on the breast and hide behind a nursing apron. But the rigmarole required for the set-up, you see, just doesn't lend itself to discretion in public.

I felt ashamed of the thing around my neck, as if I was a deficient mother for not having sufficient breast milk. I feared it made me look like some mommy monstrosity. I found myself looking on with envy as other moms clutched their babies to their breasts at the first whimper, while I had to fiddle with my albatross of an upside-down bottle to my son's impatient cries. I daydreamed about easy breastfeeding as I showered away the residue of even the best cloth tape from my sticky nipples.

One night, our child momentarily stopped breathing. He turned out to be just fine, but as nervous first-time parents, we called 911 and the paramedics took us to the nearest hospital. I readied the SNS in the ambulance, and my one-month-young son and I were wheeled into the emergency room to gasps of "aw" from the medical staff. Surely, the concern in their eyes was for my boy, but I couldn't help feeling that they also were judging me. His mouth was still coupled to my breast, just finishing a few last gulps of formula from the dangling bottle.

Or, there was the time when my husband frantically tried to hang baby blankets over the car windows while I removed my blouse and nursed from the backseat of our meter-parked car outside a dim sum restaurant in Chinatown. He scrambled from window to window, unwittingly drawing sidewalk glances, as the automated controls chewed up the blankets or, if the opening was too wide, the blankets slid right down again. Yet another time, we retreated to the women's room of a tony West Los Angeles café; my husband changed the baby's diaper while I taped up; and then I squeezed baby and self onto the top shelf of a low bookcase in the restroom, feet resting upon the toilet for support, while our son drank his fill. My husband, too embarrassed to be seen leaving the women's room alone, waited for the feeding to be over. Twenty minutes later, we emerged triumphant from the restroom only to meet the frowning faces of the line formed outside.

Cumbersome as it was, something compelled me to keep using the SNS, day after night and night after day. Maybe it was the comfort of knowing that my baby was taking in some of the benefits of breast milk with each feed; perhaps it was the satisfaction of seeing my milk supply grow; surely it was the joy of watching my son collapse into a sated sleep between my breasts after each nursing.

All the effort was worth it in the end. After four months, I was producing enough milk on my own that I only needed the SNS for every other feeding. By the time our son reached his sixth month and I returned to work, I was able to reduce use of the SNS to once in the morning and once before bed. I had sufficient milk for the other feedings, including what I pumped at the office. Midway into month ten, our family went abroad for three months, and I finally abandoned both the bottle around my neck and the pump. Although my milk was never abundant, I produced enough to supplement solids through the first thirteen months. Perhaps, I did really beat the odds. In the process, those initials of SNS took on a new meaning: through "*slow-n-s*teady" persistence, I gave my son breast milk.

PLANES, HOTELS AND CONFERENCE ROOMS: A PUMPING ADVENTURE

ALLISON LEWINSON

P RIOR TO HAVING MY FIRST CHILD, Emma, I was determined to breastfeed. I knew that breastfeeding while working full-time would not be easy, but I was psyched and ready to tackle that challenge. However, during my pregnancy, I had no idea how early on my will as a mother would be tested. After an extremely complicated delivery, I was in the ICU for the first three days of Emma's life, which meant I was unable to start breastfeeding. Emma was on formula and loving it. On day four, I was back in post-delivery and doing well. The head of lactation came in and was beyond thrilled to find out that I was very much on-board to try whatever it took to start breastfeeding. The lactation nurse set me up—I had bottles connected to tiny tubes that were taped to my chest and extended to my nipples so that when Emma latched onto my boob, she would still get the beloved formula, but also, hopefully, some breast milk. Lucky for me, it worked! I learned that my daughter loved any kind of "dairy-like" substance—formula or breast milk, she'll take whatever and even today she loves the taste of milk, no matter what kind or percentage (score!). Amazingly, I started to produce a steady supply of colostrum just like it was hour one—what a feat! Rather than feeling defeated and exhausted, this experience left me even more motivated to continue breastfeeding until I met my goal.

Along with the bottle/tube contraption, the head of lactation also brought in the hospital-grade pump and directed me to pump in-between feedings. Feeding, pumping, feeding, pumping, in the hospital and then at home. Fortunately, after the first few days at home I was able to wean off the bottle/tube contraption and rely solely on my breasts. I enjoyed breastfeeding—there was no planning, prep or clean-up involved, I would just pick up my daughter, stick her on my boob and she was happy. Although I still got extremely sore nipples, some cracking, and a lot of pain, I was so determined for my daughter to have 100 percent breast milk as long as I could produce it. This was something I was able to control and after the complications of delivery and dealing with this miracle-of-life baby that was now mine, my ability to control what my daughter ate was a huge comfort to me.

I had read that my milk supply would only get stronger with the more times I fed or pumped and I'd been advised to take advantage of the first few months, when my sole focus was on feeding my child. I worked hard to build up a supply of milk I could freeze. This became a game in my head, where the more milk I froze, the more I was winning. I had no idea how long I would breastfeed, so this gave me solace that whenever my milk supply did dry up, I would still be able to give my baby breast milk for a little longer. Of course, the frozen breast milk still had an expiration date, but it was five months out, giving me time to keep the frozen supply steady when I ended up taking from my treasured stash.

When my daughter was five months old, I started back at work. I was extremely fortunate that I worked from home the majority of the time, but I still had to travel to the San Francisco for our annual conference, a conference that lasted four days. To make matters worse, that year my company added on an extra two-day conference for my group, prior to the annual conference. I was dreading this conference and I could not muster up the courage to let my manager know I would not be able to attend. I was determined to make this work. It may sound terrible, but as much as I was going to miss being with my baby, all I could think about was how I was going to get through this conference, continue to pump, and keep EVERY drop of milk I produced. I knew my baby would be safe and well-loved while I was away (perhaps I could sleep through the night!), but how was I logistically going to save my milk and transport it back to my home in Los Angeles?

The hotel was no problem: I reserved a refrigerator. The conference was not as easy, but new mothers would be able to pump in the first aid room at the conference center. I had my trusty Medela black freezer bag to move the milk from the conference first aid room back to my hotel at the end of each day. I was like a chicken with its head cut off, running around the huge conference center back and forth to the first aid room when I needed to pump, but I was determined. Now ... how was I going to bring all the milk on the plane? This was not so straightforward. Prior to the trip, I researched online ... not much help. I read a suggestion that with dry ice, my milk could keep while going through the airport and on the plane. Lovely. Where was I going to get dry ice? And if I could find a place that sold it, how was I going to have time to get it right before going to the airport? Nope, not going to work. Of course, this was only a few years ago, so no more than three-ounce bottles of liquid fitting into a quart-size bag were allowed on the plane. That, along with hearing the horror story of a woman having to dump all her milk going through security, oh boy, what to do?

The pre-conference started on a Saturday, so I had my husband and baby come with me for the weekend. They left Monday morning and I just had to get through until Thursday night. By Thursday night, my Medela bag was filled to the rim with milk bags and then some. I froze a couple of freezer-pack bags and triple-bagged everything using the hotel laundry bags. At the airport, I weighed the risk of getting caught with so much milk and having to dump it and decided to shove the milk bags in my suitcase and check it, not taking a chance. Luckily it was only an hour flight ... sure enough the milk survived and I was safe back at home with my baby. Phew ... first trip—success! Over the next few months, I had a few day trips from LA to San Francisco and another conference in Las Vegas. No problem; I had my portable pump in tow. I now had my newfound discovery, pump bags that taped to the pump so there was no pouring of milk from bottle to bag, including no bottles to clean. I also had my system down of the on-the-go pump wipes along with my travel Babyganics bottle cleaner and tiny brush. My hotel bathroom became my kitchen sink and drying rack. I was prepared, ready for my next day trip to the Bay Area. I scheduled the trip to leave on the 6:00 a.m. flight and return on the 4:00 p.m. flight—just enough time to get to the office early, pump, attend my meeting, and get back to the airport to pump again before my flight took off. At this point, pumping in the bathroom became a good option. The idea of it grossed me out, but I hung everything from the coat hook in the stall and maneuvered so as to not touch anything by keeping extra napkins in-hand.

Since it was a day trip, all I brought was my portable pump backpack and my laptop bag. I rushed off the plane to meet my co-workers and headed out to grab a taxi. Standing in the taxi line with my male co-workers, all of a sudden I gasped. Loudly. "Oh my gosh, I left my pump on the plane!" I ran back to the airline office, praying the plane had not taken off. What would I do if it had? There was no way I could go the whole day without pumping—my breasts would burst! I would have to miss the meeting and take a taxi to find a store and buy a new pump. The whole trip would be a disaster. My heart leaped when the airline worker informed me that the plane was still at the gate and they had my bag and an airport attendant would bring it to baggage claim. PHEW! Now I just had to get over my embarrassment of the scene I made in front of the account executive and regional vice president male colleagues I was with. Fortunately, the vice president clearly remembered helping his wife during the pumping and breastfeeding with their daughter, so he understood my reaction.

The two colleagues I was traveling with had to go ahead to ensure they made the meeting on time, so I grabbed my own taxi. At this point, there would be no time to pump before the meeting once I got to the office. The only option, in my mind, was to pump *in* the taxi. Fortunate again, the taxi driver was a very sweet father and very respectful. I used my "hooter-hider" cover and my portable battery and sat back in the seat while we drove in to the city. By the time we got to the office, all I had to do was drop my milk off at the refrigerator and I was set.

My focus and determination to feed my daughter breastmilk lasted just shy of a year. From working to produce breastmilk several days after my daughter was born to continuing to pump when the environment and circumstances made it so difficult, I learned that if I really want something and I focus, I can overcome feats I would have deemed impossible.

WHEN A BODY FEEDS A BODY: REFLECTIONS ON BREASTFEEDING

CARRIE SNYDER

MY BREASTFEEDING YEARS: so straightforward, so simple on the mother/child continuum, when a warm boob offering milk could answer virtually every need. Hungry? Breast. Fussy? Squirmy? Tired? Breast. Unknown existential angst? But of course: breast. The only thing my breasts couldn't do was change a diaper.

My husband had to invent and maintain a roster of soothing techniques, but I was a one-note performer singing a one-note song; and what a seductive song it was, for both me and my children.

It must have been; only now, from my new perspective of relative freedom, can I reflect on the sacrifices inherent in the nursing relationship.

For nearly a decade, and until very recently, I was a lactating and/or pregnant woman. For nearly a decade, therefore, my hips housed and cradled growing foreign bodies till they were ready to be squeezed out and fed by breast, for many months, and even years. Our first child refused solid food till he was eight months old, and did not drink from a bottle or a cup till he was nearly a year. I was pregnant again, and my milk dried up, and I thought he might perish of thirst; but it turned out that he was perfectly capable of cup-management, and likely had been for some time. How could I have known he'd been making an aesthetic rather than a necessary choice? He was my first.

Every lactating mother has a comical and humiliating nursing story. Here's my best. On my inaugural outing to a public venue with my first-born, who was, as they say, "colicky," he was three weeks old, awake, and frantically squalling. We were seated at a small table in a crowded café and I can't even describe how much I wanted to take a bite of my curried tuna sandwich on freshly baked olive bread. Even then, utter mothering novice, I grasped the only answer to the dilemma: still unused to whipping out a nipple amidst strangers, I fumbled with the multiple hooks and buttons of my "breastfeeding-friendly" bra and shirt till at last I managed to stuff his indignant little face hurriedly atop the fulsome, exposed breast. In regular life, I am a flat-chested woman. When lactating, I swell several cup sizes and produce enough milk to feed a café filled with screaming babies. But my babe was past soothing by breast. Instead of latching on, he arched away, and I stared in horror as a shot of highly-pressurized milk squirted past a patron's head and splattered the glass of a nearby window. It was like a weapon firing. Needless to say, I got the sandwich to go.

I've choked all of my babies with too much milk. I hope that won't turn out to be a metaphor for something.

If you've never breastfed, but are contemplating doing so, skip this part. Here is where we learn that breastfeeding does not occur at regular and manageable four-hour intervals. Here is where we reveal that breastfeeding your infant is a non-stop event, and that the first several months post-birth will fade instantly into a vapour of sleep-deprivation and squishy incoherence. Everything you own will smell faintly of sour milk and baby's barf (not such a bad scent, by the way). Your t-shirts will sport round stains where a breast, pad forgotten, has leaked; the stains will prove permanent, which probably is a metaphor for something. You will wake multiple times each night to feed your baby, to stop him from crying, or because he is hungry, or because you absolutely and desperately crave immediate return to sleep *and you don't know what else to do.*

I've milked myself over a hotel sink, in an attempt to clear a painfully blocked duct before dressing up to attend a family reunion. (Blocked ducts and infections seem to pop up at the worst times, such as moments before being due to host a sit-down meal for twenty.) I've sat in quiet rooms alone with a distractable baby, hearing adults talk and laugh on the other side of the door; sometimes, I've felt left out and lonely; but other times, I've felt comforted by this fleeting time alone with my ever-growing child. I've learned the best foods to eat while simultaneously nursing; and concurrent with that, the best foods to cook (nothing with hot drippy liquid: take note). I've read thousands of picture books to toddlers while nursing, and watched far more reality television than is strictly advisable while my infant nursed and nursed and nursed in the gentle hours of the evening. I even mastered the art of breastfeeding a baby in a sling while pushing a double stroller.

And let me tell you, I loved it all.

In many ways, breastfeeding is a template for parenthood: by turns embarrassing, painful, blissful, and, inevitably, a unique ever-changing process. You will swing between having too much to give, and not enough, between taking pleasure in the giving, and feeling impatient, between yearning for this stage never to end and wishing it were over.

Now it is over. I will never lactate again. My last little nurser was talking by the time we gave it up, and he complained about the dwindling supply: "No milk in there, mama!" he would say, taking an exploratory sip and then proceeding to squeeze the nipple. I let this go on rather longer than you might think sane, but we finally said goodbye.

"All done the boobie," we said.

I miss it. But I'm not nostalgic, exactly. I'm grateful. I'm grateful that my body could be of such profound usefulness to another. But I'm also grateful for the renewed energy my body has experienced post-lactation. I know my body differently, now. I know that it has astonishing capabilities and strengths, but I also know that it has limitations that are quite beyond my thinking mind. My body continues to remind me, quietly, that it can nourish life in other ways, feed and comfort and protect and honour. For this time, here on earth, my body is lit with spirit. It is a home; and everyone must leave home in one way or another, perhaps many times during the span of a life.

My body knew that we were tapering off. It quietly slowed production. And in the end, the transition was painless. The last time we breastfed together, my littlest was worn out after a busy morning and he asked to nurse, a rare request, and he lay in my arms like he hadn't done for many months, relaxing into unexpected sleep. Though he was sucking on an essentially empty breast, he did not object; nor did I. I held him until he was perfectly soothed, as if he'd reverted to infancy just for this last occasion, till finally, I pulled him off the breast and covered him with a blanket on the couch.

We were done.

THE PRICE OF A BOOB'S JOB

MARIA POLONCHEK

ABOUT FIVE YEARS AGO, when my twin sons were newborns, I found myself at the lake, in a bikini, sitting next to a skinny blond from Florida with fake tits. One could argue that we had the best-looking racks at the lake: both of us had boobs that were big, round, and firm. Firm is an understatement; they were hard as rocks, really. And they rested high enough that we could both probably lower our chins to take a nap. I should have been proud that my free, real breasts looked just as good as her three-thousand-dollar fake breasts. But the milk leaking out of my bathing suit and dripping onto my leg reminded me that, while hers would still look like they do in a year, I would be tucking mine into my pants.

That summer I had become a mother which meant, as Rebecca Woolf articulates so well in her memoir *Rockabye*, my pussy had become a vagina and my tits had turned into breasts. It was Fourth of July and there were going to be fireworks over the lake, but we were heading home early that year: my husband, Chris, and I were not getting along because he couldn't tell the blonde had fake tits. I had to explain to him how one could identify them, which infuriated me. How could he not tell? How could this shallow, self-absorbed, superficial woman get by in life with fake tits passing as real ones? How was I supposed to celebrate freedom with her around?

The weekend trip to a friend's lake house was not going well. I sprayed milk in Chris's face in the car on the way down because he was mocking Tori Amos. He didn't think it was funny.

131

Then I met a colleague of my husband's, Matt, a handsome guy in his early twenties, and got a much-needed boost to my confidence when he turned his attention to me until he asked, "So, are you like, lactating *right now?*"

Although I am crazy-in-love with my husband, I felt a pang inside when I realized a guy with whom I might have been flirting wildly a few years prior was asking what it felt like when my milk came in. What a strange obsession this guy had with a woman's biological functioning. For the rest of the weekend, Matt wanted to be the one who introduced me to newcomers. "This is Maria," he'd say. "She's lactating."

And then we had the blonde from Florida. When she arrived, she stepped out of a luxury rental car in heels and designer sunglasses, her dark bronze skin seeming even more exotic against her white dress. Along with the men, I sized up her long legs, unnaturally large breasts considering her otherwise small frame, and was immediately relieved to see her. As soon as she spoke, I knew I wouldn't like her, but she would definitely help me fit in with the other women. If one thing can unify a group of otherwise hesitant females, it's a rich bimbo with fake tits. The rest of us would congregate in the water on floaties, out of range, and talk about her and her boob job and bad personality and try to feel better that at least we were interesting people.

Naturally, I had to know what Chris thought of her breasts. When we were alone the first night, I managed to manipulate the conversation enough to get the information I wanted. (He eventually learned how to avoid my "traps," as he presently refers to them.) I wasn't upset when he admitted she had a nice body, but I was outraged at his genuine surprise to learn her breasts were fake.

"How can you think they're real?" I asked him, incredulously. "They don't move when she does, they're incredibly high and far apart, and that hot-pink string bikini does not provide the kind of support she would *really* need to lift a rack like that!"

He was silent for a moment, which lead me to believe that he was about to give in and admit, *You're right, Maria. Of course her breasts are fake. How could I have not realized it? She is obviously insecure and shallow and half the woman you are.* Instead, he replied, "Do you realize you've been looking at her chest more than any guy here?"

Chris and I had to do a lot of recalibrating those first couple years after becoming parents. In another life, details from a weekend at the lake included tequila, pot, and sunburns. The transition to breastmilk, diapers, and shade wasn't an easy one. We were among the first of our friends to have children and we were struggling. Looking back, I view that weekend as a clumsy attempt to fit our new life back into our old one. It wasn't working. Why did I think it would? Didn't I learn anything by witnessing Brittney Spears' complete and utter disaster of a transition? And she had personal assistants.

In the early days after becoming a mother I felt as if I was living in an alternate, invisible world. The first time I left the house alone after nesting in with my new family was sometime during the second week. I was excited by the prospect of getting out by myself, even if it was just to drop something off at the post office. As I was solely responsible for producing the boys' food, my husband was nervous for me to leave without giving him a back-up supply of breast milk. I pumped for fifteen minutes to leave the house for ten, and went on my way. As I stood in the same-old post office line with the usual suspects clutching their parcels and sighing, I started to fidget with anxiety. Had life always been this mundane previous to the delivery of my twins? I suddenly became overwhelmed with an urge to grab the nearest pedestrian and start shaking him. "DO YOU REALIZE I HAVE GIVEN BIRTH TO ANOTHER HUMAN BEING?" I wanted to yell. "DOES ANYONE HERE HAVE ANY FUCKING CLUE WHAT THAT MEANS?"

And now, after having a third, I still can't get over the enormous depths of meaning and intensity having children has given my life. But that doesn't mean I can't also be shallow. I will admit now to a superficial realization I've had since being twice pregnant and breastfeeding three children: I used to have spectacular tits. Perfect, really. I still blush when I remember a decade-old scene, when I was single and a new lover was seeing me naked for the first time. His expression. And he tried to play it cool. "I bet you hear this all the time," he said. "But I have to say, you have amazing breasts."

And I did, though I didn't realize it at the time. Back then, I was modest and embarrassed. I'd had a difficult rapport with my breasts. I spent the majority of my post-adolescent life hating them. To the girls in my junior high and high school, plump, perky breasts signaled "loose" behavior. I couldn't erase all of the "slut" graffiti next to my name in the bathroom stalls, which was in no way an assessment of my sexual activity as much as it was determined by my 34C bra size. (In retrospect, now that I've worn nursing bras in size DD, I'm wondering why a C was considered so big…)

After high school, once I got more serious about running and lifting weights, I was told a number of times, in various ways, that "real" athletes don't have breasts. They are just mounds of fat, after all. These comments, on top of the names that accumulated over the years ("Booby-diver," from the days at the swimming pool, particularly stings), were thrown into one big pile in my mind under, "Reasons Why I Hate My Boobs." I spent most of those years hiding my breasts, smashing them, covering them, despising them. I used to cup them with my hands in front of the mirror and press up as hard as I could to admire my ribs underneath; what I might look like if my breasts weren't there.

After so much ambivalence over my breasts, when it was time to breastfeed, I was ready to let them shine. Because formula was so popular for so many years, I've heard other women say they grew up not knowing milk could be found somewhere other than a bottle. For me, it was the opposite. My mother breastfed all five of her children. If I saw a baby with a bottle, the child was a toddler drinking juice. I grew up thinking formula was an emergency-only solution for babies who were adopted. My mother-in-law breastfed Chris and his two younger sisters as well, so he was not shy about the process. Now that I understand more about birthing, feeding, and scheduling, I realize there are as many styles and choices for parenting as there are shapes and sizes of breasts, but for me, breastfeeding was not optional. Finally, I thought, after so many years of being unsure about my body, these breasts are going to enable me to do something natural and healthy and I would love them for it. I assumed breastfeeding would come easily and that I might even have moments of euphoria I've heard described by other mothers. Even when I found out I was having twins, when people *really* started to question my decision, I didn't think twice. Two boobies, two babies, right? I couldn't get more efficient if I tried.

I was not ready for the phenomenon that is "over-production." When my milk came in, I didn't have the typical couple of days of uncomfortable fullness: I had weeks, months. It didn't matter how many breast pads I used to absorb the leaking, how many cabbage leaves I stuffed down my shirt. Within minutes of nursing or pumping, sticky white liquid would spray from all ducts. It would squirt the boys in the face, as soon as I pulled down my nursing bra. Latching on wasn't a problem, as they just had to open their tiny mouths and lap it up with their tongues, like little puppies drinking from a big bowl.

With two babies eating every couple of hours, I was nursing over eight hours a day. The fabric on our couch wore down into a particular round pattern where I sat day and night with my twin-breast-feeding pillow in what my brother referred to as the "double-barrel position." When I realized how often I was taking off my shirt, I stopped dressing altogether. After several baby-gift deliveries, the UPS man was no longer surprised when I answered the door in my underwear, an oversized U-shaped pillow fastened around my waste, with an infant on my boob. Chris had grown accustomed to the sight of me plugged into the auxiliary jack in our car, pumping on the Interstate as we passed semi-drivers and police officers alike. The extra supply finally straightened itself out after six long months, when I decided to supplement one feeding a day with organic formula. At nine months, I gave the boys half of their feedings with formula and discovered what it might have been like to be producing milk for only one baby.

But even when I had only one baby, my third, the over-production picked up where it had left off. After my daughter was born, I had the same problems I had with the twins, including plugged ducts and mastitis, until several months in, as a last resort, I took some estrogen pills to lighten my supply. I never did come to enjoy breastfeeding like I thought I would—an experience I thought would be natural and easy until I actually went through it.

I can't help but feel I've always been disappointed by my breasts. They used to be a source of anxiety, aesthetically. Then they were a source of anxiety, pragmatically. And now that they resemble what my friend Alix refers to as tennis balls hanging in the bottom of tube socks, they are a source of anxiety again. I'm so worried about looking like I belong on the cover of *National Geographic* with the tribal women that I can't possibly have a realistic grasp of what condition my boobs are in. How much more unappreciative can a woman get when her breasts have done their biologically fundamental job *three times over* and she can't learn to accept them for what they are?

There is a big lie I tell myself often: that I don't care about physical appearances. I don't care how I look, how others look, and how we compare. And as I was floating in the lake with the other women that Fourth of July weekend, scrutinizing the blonde from Florida, and then scrutinizing ourselves, I said something that I hope I believed, even if it was just for a moment. I told the girls that creating, and then growing, birthing, and feeding another human being has made this "body stuff" unimportant. When we discover what our bodies are capable of—and childbirth taught me that it's beyond what I ever could imagine—there is no choice other than to be reverent of what we have, even if it's not always our idea of "perfect."

But, yes, I care how I look. And I *really* care that I care. I'm not proud of considering the possibility that one day, I may call the skinny blonde from Florida for the number of her plastic surgeon. For now, I am wearing my extra-separating, extra-lifting, extra-uncomfortable Miracle Bra from Victoria's Secret. But that doesn't mean that I'm not also proud of my breasts from the past. Proud of how they once looked. Proud of nourishment they once provided. And I hope to learn from women who are proud of their own breasts now: breasts that are breastfeeding; breast that are embarrassingly small or overwhelmingly large; breasts that have been through a thing or two. These are women who know that payment for a boob's job is more than a matter of money.

CONTRIBUTOR NOTES

Rachel Epp Buller (editor) is a feminist-art historian-printmaker-mama of three whose engagement with breastfeeding in all of these roles is best summed up by the time she nursed, sitting on a curb, while wearing graduation robes in 100-degree weather. Her most recent books are *Reconciling Art and Mothering* (Ashgate, 2012) and *Mothering Mennonite,* co-edited with Kerry Fast (Demeter, 2013).

Anna Braff is a first-time mommy and lawyer. She lives with her husband, their son, and two dogs by the beach in Los Angeles. She enjoys spending time with her beautiful family and friends, traveling, sleeping, going to the beach, and playing volleyball.

Sarah Campbell once was a stay-at-home mom who loved, survived and now misses the time spent nursing her children. She writes short stories, reads more books than the library where she works likes to put on hold, and enjoys every moment she gets with her wonderful husband in Waterloo, Ontario.

Adriann Cocker, a native of Los Angeles, is fascinated by the everyday world and attempts to shine a light on our true selves by sharing these stories—both at work in Consumer Insights, and at play in a blog about loft-life and family in downtown LA. Adriann also enjoys traveling with her young son and scouting for her husband's urban photography.

Mandy Cohen is a wife, a mom and a TV producer. Once a week, she tears herself away from her family and travels to produce a live sporting event for ESPN. Breastfeeding and traveling was one of the hardest yet most rewarding things she has ever done.

Vanessa Druckman is a freelance writer and blogger living in Chicago with her husband and four children. As her family has grown, Vanessa has come to think of breast milk as the first step in raising adventurous eaters. When her son renamed her breasts the boobie milk makers, she knew her transformation into a nursing mom was complete.

Norine Dworkin-McDaniel created the illustrated humor blog Science of Parenthood (www.scienceofparenthood.com) and serves as its Chief of Scientific Snarkiness. When she's not blogging about the endless mysteries of parenting an active, inquisitive seven-year-old boy at Don't Put Lizards In Your Ears (www.norinedworkin.com/blog) and Lifescript's Parent Talk blog (www.lifescript.com), she works as a freelance writer. Her articles have appeared in *More, Health, Parents, American Baby, iVillage, Family Circle, Redbook, Readers Digest, Prevention, Marie Claire, All You* and *WhatToExpect.com*. She's at work on a collection of humor essays about being a late-in-life mom.

Gina Kaysen Fernandes lives in the greater Los Angeles region with her husband and two sons. She enjoys cooking, gardening and building sandcastles at the beach. When she's not hanging out with family, Gina is an award-winning documentary producer, writer and PR consultant. Her passion for storytelling began when she worked as a journalist and TV news producer in the Northwest.

Micala Gingrich-Gaylord is a Kansas native. She studied painting and sculpture at the University of Kansas and now pays for rent and food with her work as Expressive Arts Center founder and director for Youthville, an organization for children and youth in secure care. She likes reading poems aloud and overthrowing the state, all while knitting, drawing and making art with her daughter, Basil.

Wendy Haldeman is a co-founder of the Pump Station & Nurtury. She received both her undergraduate and master's degree in nursing at UCLA. Wendy is an International Board Certified Lactation Consultant (IBCLC), and a certified Happiest Baby on the Block instructor. She lectures frequently on human lactation at medical and nursing schools and has been identified by publications, such as Fit Pregnancy, as an "expert" in her field. At The Pump Station, Wendy teaches a number of classes including prenatal breastfeeding, newborn infant care, working without weaning and a class for new grandparents. She and her husband Tim are proud of their two grown daughters and adore their two granddaughters. When not working, Wendy loves spending time with her family and friends, is an avid reader, and enjoys hiking.

Jessica Claire Haney is a freelance writer and mother of two living in Northern Virginia. Her writing has appeared in *Mothering, Hip Mama, The Washington Post, Journal of Attachment Parenting International,* the anthology *From the Heart, TheDCMoms.com* and *The Washington Times Communities Online.* She founded and co-leads a local chapter of Holistic Moms Network and is working on her first novel. Her website is JessicaClaireHaney.com, and her blog is Crunchy-ChewyMama.com.

Corky Harvey, MS, RN, IBCLC, is the co-founder of The Pump Station & Nurtury, the first new parent resource center of its kind. She is a registered nurse with a Master's degree in maternal/newborn nursing from the University of Maryland. She is an International Board Certified Lactation Consultant, a certified Happiest Baby on the Block educator, and was a long-time Childbirth Educator. Corky does one-on-one lactation consultations, teaches Prenatal Breastfeeding, Baby Care, and new Grandparents classes. One of her favorite things to do is facilitate the New Mothers Breastfeeding Support Groups. She was on the faculty of the UCLA Lactation Educator and Consultant programs for many years and still lectures at hospitals, conferences and parent venues. Corky has three grown children who were breastfed and she loves to claim that their intelligence is linked to this. In her spare time she enjoys traveling with her husband Dean, especially to Germany where her two darling grandsons live. She loves to sing, and is a member of an International championship women's barbershop chorus.

Juleigh Howard-Hobson squeezes writing into the brouhaha that is her life. Her kid-centric work has appeared in *Nesting: It's a Chick Thing* (Workman), *Bare Your Soul* (Seal Press), *Chick Ink* (Adams Media), *The Girls Book of Success* (Little, Brown), *Hip Mama Magazine, Home Education Magazine, Errant Parent* and other places.

Aleria Jensen's poems and essays have been published in journals such as *Orion Magazine, Literary Mama, Potomac Review,* and Terrain.org. Her work can be found in the anthology *Wonder and Other Survival Skills* and in *Wildbranch: An Anthology of Nature, Environmental, and Place-based Writing.* She lives in Juneau, Alaska with her partner and their two children.

Caryn Leschen is a cartoonist, illustrator, writer and graphic designer, best known for her advice comic, Ask Aunt Violet, and her persistent appearance in the *Wimmin's Comix* and *Twisted Sisters* anthologies. Coming up next will be an Ask Aunt Violet collection and a graphic novel, *Miss Internal*

Revenue. Caryn grew up in Queens, New York, but lives in San Francisco where she teaches digital animation, illustration and writing at the University of San Francisco.

Allison Lewinson lives in Newport Beach, CA, with her husband Matt, daughter Emma and their dog Charlie. She works full-time for a hi-tech company as a Customer Success Manager. When not working, she is having a blast watching her toddler learn new things every day. She loves spending time as a family and with their extended family—eating, playing and being silly. Since becoming a mom, Allison is now obsessed with *listening* to books on her iPhone—able to rapidly finish several books on the road, her favorite (or easiest) way to de-stress.

Lacy Lynn is a self-proclaimed public health advocate and is studying to become a breastfeeding peer counselor. In her free time she works on her website, ubermotherrunner.com, to create an experience-based resource for prenatal, postpartum and breastfeeding mother runners. She is passionate about encouraging others to learn what "inspire yourself" means.

Elizabeth Lyons is an author, designer, humorist, mother of five, on-call plumber, chauffeur, virgin organic gardener, DIY addict, Anthropologie lover, hostage negotiator, and guitar student. One thing she is *not* is any sort of Superwoman. She simply demands the right to do things her way—a way that often defies even the most creative imaginations—and she strives to inspire others to do things *their* way (once she helps them figure out what their way is). Elizabeth lives in Arizona with her five kids, three dogs, two fish (RIP Cosmo and Paul), four barely surviving organic gardens, and whatever (or whomever) else has taken up residence with them in the last five minutes.

Jenna McCarthy is an internationally published writer, TED-speaker, former radio personality and the author of five books including *If It Was Easy They'd Call the Whole Damn Thing a Honeymoon: Living with and Loving the TV-Addicted, Sex-Obsessed, Not-so-handy Man You Married.* Her work has appeared in more than 60 magazines, on dozens of web sites and in several anthologies including the popular *Chicken Soup* series. An insomniac and self-confessed social media addict, Jenna tweets, posts and blogs obsessively. You can find out how she survived tanorexia and watch the hilarious trailer for her latest book at www.jennamccarthy.com.

Mosa Maxwell-Smith is a storyteller and improviser living and writing in Oakland, California. In the past she has done everything from teaching fourth grade to working at a pole-dance studio. She now spends much of her time chasing a busy preschooler and bemoaning the loss of her amazing nursing-era cleavage. Find Mosa at boobjuice.wordpress.com.

Jill Neumann is a writer, among other things. She is a featured blogger at 5cities6women.com. She spends her time eating, laughing, watching bad TV, eating more, and writing about the little things. Jill lives in Chicago with her daughter, who is by far the best thing she has ever done.

Ama Christabel Nsiah-Buadi is a writer and journalist whose work has aired on NPR, the BBC, the Canadian Broadcasting Corporation and the Pacifica Network. She's the founder of Awesome Little Beings (awesomelittlebeings.com), a multimedia storytime series featuring stories from all over the world. She's also the proud mother of Abena, a smart, funny girl with powerful lungs.

Kari O'Driscoll is a writer who lives in the Pacific Northwest with her husband, two children, one dog, one cat, and one hamster. She has written for *BuddhaChickLife* magazine and *The Cancer Poetry Project*, writes book reviews for *Bookplea-*

sures.com and has a blog at www.the-writing-life.blogspot. com where she writes about parenting, philosophy, cooking, social justice, health issues and anything else that strikes her fancy. Her daughters are a tiny bit mortified that she wrote this frankly, but someday they will appreciate it.

Eliana Osborn is a writer, mother and professor living in the desert southwest. She has published work in *Dash, Blood and Thunder, Segullah, Noah, Literary Mama, The Mom Egg, Hip Mama,* and a variety of commercial magazines.

Sarah Pinneo is the author of *Julia's Child* (Plume 2012), a comedic novel of motherhood and food. Her work has appeared in *The New York Times* and *Boston Globe Magazine,* among other publications. Visit her at www.SarahPinneo.com.

Maria Polonchek is a Kansas native living in the Bay Area. She calls herself a writer, though three young children at home have slowed productive output. Her essays have appeared in *Brain, Child,* and she is currently working on her first novel.

Amanda Rosen-Prinz is a writer and currently lactating mother. Her experiences with breastfeeding inspired her to become a Lactation Educator Counselor to help other mothers through their breastfeeding struggles. She lives in Los Angeles with her husband and their two children.

Rochelle Jewel Shapiro is the author of *Miriam the Medium* (Simon and Schuster) and *Kaylee's Ghost* (Amazon). She's a professional psychic who has published in NYT (Lives), *Newsweek* (My Turn) and in many magazines and anthologies. She teaches writing at UCLA Extension. http://rochellejewelshapiro.com.

Jennifer Andrau Shpilsky is a freelance non-fiction writer and advocate for environmental health issues. Jennifer drew early inspiration for her literary work while residing in Moscow, Russia. There she worked for MAIK Nauka/Interperiodica in cooperation with Pleiades Publishing editing scientific journals in support of the Russian Academy of Sciences. Jennifer also was a health contributor for the American Medical Center of Kyiv, Ukraine magazine *To Your Health*. She currently lives in Los Angeles with her husband and two children where she is working toward her master's degree in Linguistics.

Anna G. Silver is a writer and historian who lives in West Los Angeles. When not playing mom, she teaches at a large research university in the West.

Carrie Snyder is the author of two books of fiction including *The Juliet Stories*, which was a finalist for the 2012 Governor General's Award. She has four children and figures she spent a solid decade either pregnant, breastfeeding, or both. It was good while it lasted. Carrie blogs as Obscure CanLit Mama.

Helen Tan is a trained accountant and a stay-at-home mum of three children and two dogs. She breastfed all of her children up to eight months. As her children are in their late teens, she is now enjoying some much deserved "Me" time pursuing her passions of writing, orchid growing, travelling and photography.

Roz Warren writes for *The New York Times* and *The Humor Times*, and for other venues from *Good Housekeeping* to *Girlfriendz*. Visit her website at www.rosalindwarren.com or connect with her on Facebook at www.facebook.com/writer rozwarren.

Beth Winegarner is an author and journalist whose work has appeared in the *New Yorker, Mother Jones, Wired*, and many

San Francisco Bay Area newspapers. She lives in the City by the Bay with her partner and daughter. For more, visit www. bethwinegarner.com.